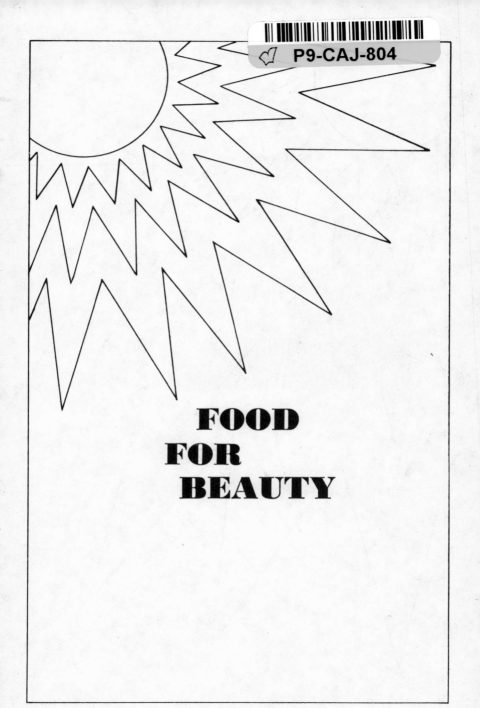

FOOD
FOR
BEAUTY

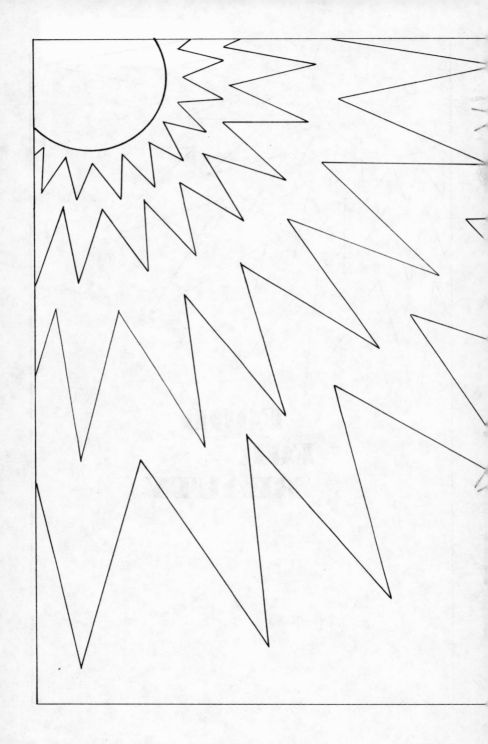

Helena Rubinstein

FOOD FOR BEAUTY

David McKay Company, Inc. | New York

Library of Congress Cataloging in Publication Data

Rubinstein, Helena, 1870-1965.
Food for beauty.

Includes index.
1. Diet. 2. Beauty, Personal. I. Title.
RA784.R8   1977   641.5′63   76-46619
ISBN 0-679-50680-2

10 9 8 7 6 5 4 3 2 1

Manufactured in the United States of America

Designed by The Etheredges

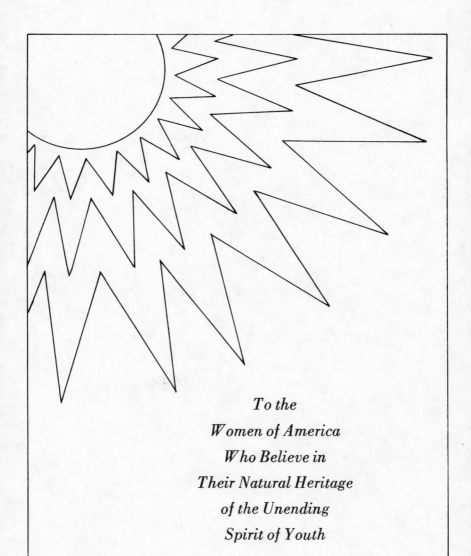

*To the
Women of America
Who Believe in
Their Natural Heritage
of the Unending
Spirit of Youth*

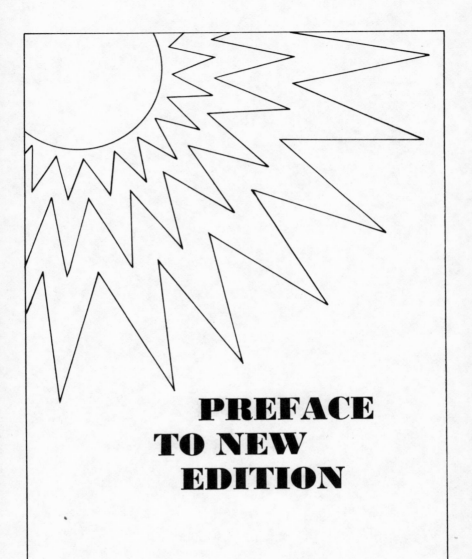

PREFACE
TO NEW
EDITION

The legendary Madame, as Helena Rubinstein was known to friends and followers, understood that a body that feels as good as it looks and is always in top form is the result of a sane and sensible diet—and one that isn't dull. She established a basic regimen for beauty, health, and lasting weight loss that is as intriguing in its culinary delights as it is astonishing in its long-range effects. But like many great men and women, Helena Rubinstein was way ahead of her time. Her sunshine nutrition diet is the forerunner of a host of diets that are popular today—including the liquid, the low carbohydrate, the high fibre, and the natural and organic diets. *Food for Beauty*, originally published in 1938, contains the only diet to incorporate the advantages of all these plans into a single overall beauty regimen—one that has won the confidence of generations of women.

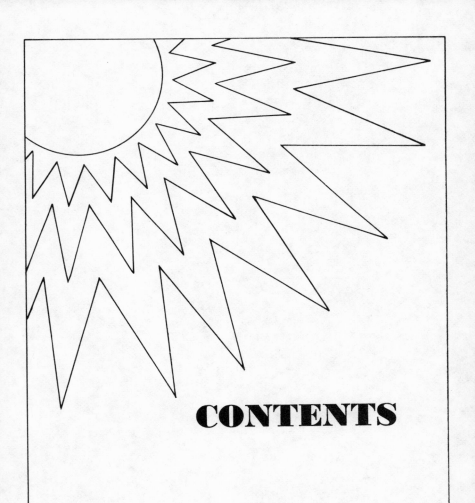

CONTENTS

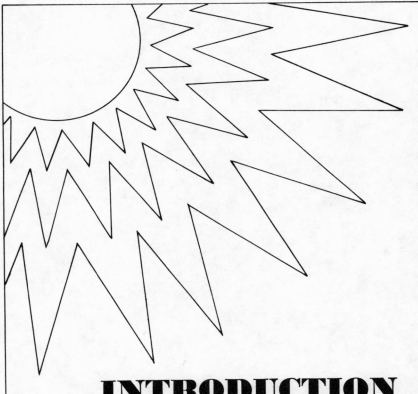

INTRODUCTION

You must be vibrant. You must be alive, active, creative in your own life, able to meet every emergency with resilience. You must be all these things to be called youthfully beautiful in these modern times. Rhythmic speed and elastic poise are the symbols of the modern woman. The satin boudoir and the ladylike "vapors" of Victorian days are no longer fashionable. Classic health is the true foundation on which every intelligent woman builds her vitality.

For years I have led a terrifically busy life. I spent

my energy without even a hint of conservation. Life everywhere demanded more exploration. The needs of countless women dragged me, tired and almost desperate for the want of rest, back and back into the study of new and ever more effective ways of making them lovelier and more cherished by the men and children they loved. Always ahead of me, I was confident, there lay some new discovery in the field of prolonging youth. I never ceased to believe with a burning faith that the conquest of beauty was like the conquest of nature. One day we shall arrive at the great secret. Then all women can achieve their heart's desire and stand fearless before their mirrors. They will be at peace with the world and themselves, for they will have become as they have dreamed of becoming.

Yes, I believed and labored in the vineyard of my own belief. But the labor finally exhausted me. Restless nights followed each other through months. No more repose. Physical refreshment became only a memory. Then abruptly I stopped. I dragged back to Paris, where I planned to undergo treatment with a famous Parisian specialist. For a time I honestly tried to follow his advice. But I saw it was not good advice—or not good enough. I suffered greater nerve tenseness; sleeplessness grew more feverish. By accident, and in a moment of frantic despair, I grasped the suggestion of a wise friend who was also a doctor. "Go to Zurich," he said. "Go there to the Bircher-Benner Sanatorium."

I must risk seeming fantastic to tell you of the joy

that came from that advice. At the world-famous health center in Zurich I saw hundreds of men and women, who had been sent there by their own doctors, eating raw fruits and vegetables, nuts and whole cereals under the watchful direction of the great Dr. Bircher-Benner.

In fact, the entire population of that beautiful city in the Alps seemed to be composed of men, women, and children who had come from the four corners of the earth to learn how to eat for health and rejuvenation. The magic words "Bircher-Benner" had enticed not only the rich but also the poor, and the place abounded in healthy children whose earliest education in eating was to insure them a long life of physical well-being.

In a few days I began to feel a surge of hope come alive again in my own body. Day after day I adhered to this *matière vivante* diet, eating all of my daily food raw in the form of fruits and vegetables. Steadily I gained vitality, poise returned to my nerves, life took on a younger hue. I completed the treatment at that amazing sanatorium in the Alps. Then I hastened back to Paris, impatient to resume my life-long habit of driving work.

Before my return to America, I spent one evening with friends in a Paris drawing room. They were astonished at my appearance. "Have you really discovered, at last, the great secret of youth?" I was asked.

My answer was, "Perhaps." At any odds, I had discovered a large part of that secret. I knew—because all my life I had been experimenting in that field—that the care of the skin with the help of scientific creams and lotions was part of the secret. And I knew, from years of observation in all my salons, that intelligently prescribed exercise is also needed for a slender charm. Yes, and for a long time I had realized that diet, too, was all-important in the great quest. But though I searched and studied for years, trying to find a diet that I could recommend without even a touch of doubt, until my Alpine experiment, I had not found the perfect diet for the beauty-hungry woman.

I was not any novice at health resorts. I think I have at one time or another, during my search for better advice to women, visited every spa, every spring, every sanatorium and cure in Europe and on this continent. Whenever I heard of a new way to health and youthful vitality, I went to its source. But at Zurich I found the ultimate answer. The exhilaration that came from my own renewed health and the recharging of my courage to go on living, inspired me to pass on this secret to other women. Nor was my own experience the only inspiration. All about me at the Bircher-Benner Sanatorium and in the streets of Zurich I saw the look of joy and thanksgiving that comes from the return of hope and the vision of youthful vitality.

Now have I answered the question that at once comes to mind when you hear that a woman in my field writes a book on food and diet? You thought beauty was my great passion. It is. But, you see, the adage "Beauty is only skin deep" is not completely true. It falls apart in the light of modern science and creative thinking. Beauty is far, far deeper than a lovely skin. A system that is clean inside as well as out, a body that is charged with health and vitality—that is the only base there is for the stream-lined glamour of the modern woman. The food you eat determines how great will be your beauty.

Now you know why I write a book on food. You know, too, why I call it *Food for Beauty*. That title is an appeal not only to your vanity. It is an appeal to every desire in your heart for *élan vitale*—that creative drive which holds off time and makes youthfulness a condition of life rather than a measure of years. But this book is more than that. It is a practical guide for healthier living in your own home. And home usually means a man and a woman and children weaving their lives together. I cannot overstate my eagerness to see entire families learn to live on raw fruits and vegetables. I have seen what it does. I want you, too, to see what it can do.

Into the preparation of this book have gone two years of study and experiment, as well as a large ex-penditure of money. I made repeated visits to Zurich, where I learned more and more about the Bircher-Benner principles of diet and the preparation of raw foods. It is really a very simple and wholesome diet of sun-blessed foods presented beautifully and served raw. In no way is it one of those starvation diets that have become the fad with misguided women who forget that health and not emaciation is the structural basis of true beauty and slenderness.

After much study in Zurich I realized that for the American taste the simplicity of the menus at the Bircher-Benner Sanatorium must be changed for a greater variety. In Europe fruits and vegetables are more expensive than they are here. Even at so renowned a health resort as Bircher-Benner's, the variety of fruits and vegetables used would seem inadequate to the American housewife of even modest income. Therefore I had to adapt the Bircher-Benner menus to the American markets, expanding their variety by adding many more luxurious fruits and berries, and extending the use of fresh vegetables to the prodigal and ever-changing bounty of our own markets and gardens.

Before writing a guide such as this, I wanted to experiment with this diet in my New York salon. Therefore I spent many thousands of dollars to open the Zurich Room, where my adaptation of the Bircher-Benner sunlight-nutrition diet could be served daily to many of the world's famous women who visit my salon for beauty advice. I knew that my experiment could not be profitable in a financial way. The Zurich Room was to be kept small, exclusive, and charming. It was not in any sense to be regarded as a restaurant. It was a laboratory for slender beauty and youthful health.

It was an expensive laboratory, yet I am satisfied with the knowledge that came out of it. All of the material in this book is based on the observations of myself and the staff physician and graduate dieticians who worked so brilliantly with me. On this diet of *matière vivante* food, on the same routine explicitly set down on the following pages, countless women (yes, and many men and children) have learned to eat for health.

But not every one could visit the Zurich Room. Distance, expense, a thousand reasons may have kept you from the pilgrimage. Yet this book will show you how to follow this great diet of sunlight food in your own home. And if it does that, I shall feel that the labor and the expense that have gone into its writing have been justified.

I wish I could stand by you and hold you to the routine. But what happened to me is proof enough that health and resilience will reward you. The fact that many of the most beautiful women in society, stars of the stage and screen, week after week, have lunched in my salon and followed this diet also in their own homes will become an inspiration to you. Ever since my girlhood in Melbourne, I have lived in Paris, London, Vienna, Warsaw, all over the civilized world, and I have replied to the whispered cries of feminine anguish with practical answers. Perhaps I have succeeded insofar as it was possible to succeed. Now I have discovered another step in that progress up toward the throne of never-aging womanhood. Your children and your husband will share the health and reawakened vitality in this diet with you. But you must persist. No classic temple was ever built overnight.

Do you need a cry of faith to urge you forward? Must you carry a banner before your eyes as you diet along the road to streamlined vitality? Then engrave these words on your woman's heart: "Health is the well from which a woman draws perpetual youth."

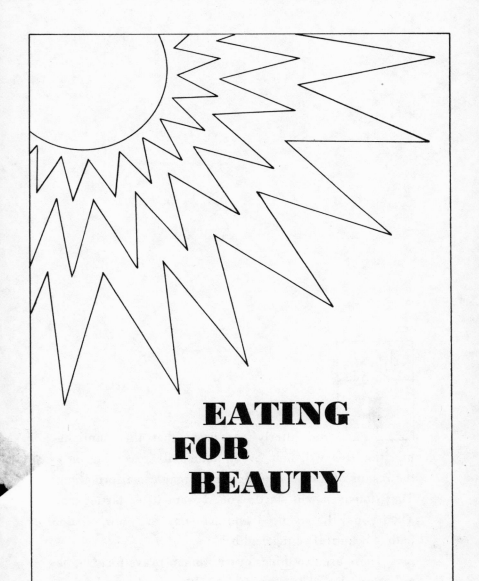

EATING
FOR
BEAUTY

I am utterly convinced that this sunlight-nutrition diet will help every human ill, excepting only the results of an accident or some organic malformation. That statement will startle you. I want it to startle you Then you will pay heed and set your feet now on the path to beautiful young health.

There are two things every woman prays for. One is a flawless skin. The other is a healthy slender body. But before she can have either, she must realize that vital cleanliness is the basis on which they are built. By vital cleanliness I mean that she must be utterly free of constipation. I mean that she can banish pills, oils, mineral salts, abdominal massage, and other temporary remedies from her day. A normally functioning system will not need such artificial aids. When she has learned to follow this beautifying diet of raw fruits and vegetables, she will discover that a properly fed body functions normally. And what does normal functioning mean in terms of beauty?

It means that the skin will be freed of blemishes. It means that sallowness, coarse pores, blackheads, and pimples will disappear. But these things cannot happen overnight. A diet of raw fruits and vegetables will achieve undreamed-of wonders. But you must continue this diet over a reasonably long period. Years of eating nothing but over-cooked foods has probably softened the muscles of your intestinal tract to such an extent that a long retoning process will be needed to give them back their natural activity.

Stated in simple terms, this diet, which will retone your intestinal system and clear your skin, requires you to eat half your daily food in the form of raw fruits and vegetables. You are not required to banish broiled or roast meats from your menu. You can even have a sweet now and then. So you see, this Food for Beauty Diet promises to transform you into a beautiful woman without making you a haggard martyr along the way.

You are surprised that I want you to eat your food raw. Yes, it must be raw and fresh and of great variety.

Bircher-Benner insists that most of your food be eaten raw. And I also insist that 50 percent of the food you eat for your beauty and health be in the natural state. That means that you can take other things after you have eaten enough raw fruits, vegetables, and nuts to comprise one half of your daily food intake. Or to reshape that definition into a rule: Select one-half of your food from the things your body needs, then select the other half from the things you feel you want terribly.

A word about the rawness of the foods in this sunlight-nutrition diet. Practically every layman believes that cooking increases the digestibility of food. That is not correct. On the contrary, in most cases, particularly where overcooking is present, the reverse is true. To the spoiled palate, to the jaded overcivilized appetite, cooking certainly does make food seem more palatable, and we therefore think cooking is a necessity for wholesome food. We forget that our gastric juices and intestinal bacteria are fully capable of making food assimilable for human needs. It may take the system a little longer to prepare and digest these raw foods, but that in no way indicates that the rawness of foods is a disadvantage. Rawness in fruits and vegetables is, on the contrary, essential for tooth health, for keeping the jaws firm and strong, for reawakening of atrophied taste perceptions, for strengthening of flabby stomach muscles— the bane of the woman who wants to keep her youthful figure—and for the general health and toning of the intestinal tract.

28

Of course, the great majority of people are accustomed to eating all of their food cooked. Their palates have become pampered and demand stimulants in the form of exciting spices and condiments. Or else their palates have grown overdelicate with the years of soft food and demand, as an unhealthful consequence, only foods that feel gentle and velvety. They cannot, or at least so many believe, stand the tonic roughness of the foods in their natural state. However, when these bad eating habits have been overcome, these same people find that in raw foods they discover new enjoyment and a surprising range of flavors.

There are other soft-food addicts who will insist that they have tried to eat raw fruits and vegetables but found them upsetting. They will tell you with all honesty that experience has proved to them that their stomach and bowels cannot stand raw food. Despite these statements made on the basis of seemingly plausible experience, their conviction about the effects of raw foods is erroneous. The scientific men at the Bircher-Benner Sanatorium in Zurich showed me literally thousands of case histories of patients cured by their raw-fruit-and-vegetable diet. Yet a large proportion of those men and women cured had insisted when they first arrived that their stomachs and intestines could not stand raw food.

The Food for Beauty Diet consists of a generous variety of raw fruits and vegetables. Not just two or three, but whenever possible, as many as five or more vegetables and fruits should be combined in a single meal. The reason for this wide variety is well founded. Fruits and vegetables, especially when served in their natural condition of ripeness and without being subjected to the chemical destruction brought about by cooking, are concentrated sources of minerals and vitamins. But each type of vegetable or fruit has its own arrangement of vitamins and supply of minerals. Each single fruit or vegetable does not contain an equal amount of all the essentials. In many cases, certain vitamins are entirely absent, but others are present in marked quantities. The variety prescribed purposefully provides more vitamins and minerals than the average individual body may need. But many bodies have special vitamin and mineral requirements. So in the safe margin offered, every individual, no matter what her particular requirements, is certain to get the maximum for her own body needs.

"Eating for beauty" becomes much more than an interesting phrase once you realize the part vitamins play in your general health and appearance. In the raw fruits and vegetables you will eat, these indispensable elements will be present to prevent disturbances to health, which in turn may cause dry skin, obstinate acne, false pigmentation, liver spots, dandruff, loss of hair, brittle fingernails, and countless other blemishes to feminine loveliness.

Let us review, briefly, some of the properties of the foods this *matière vivante* diet is based on. Carrots, pars-

30

ley, and other green vegetables will supply you with Vitamin A. Vitamin A is important in preventing drying of the skin and aids greatly in promoting normal growth.

Nuts, which are used a great deal in this diet, and the whole-grain cereals which are recommended, contain Vitamin B. Vitamin B reacts favorably on the nervous system, an important function in these times of excessive tension. B also aids in the prevention of rheumatism.

Lemons, oranges, grapefruit, strawberries, watermelon, tomato juice, watercress, cabbage, and the familiar salad greens are rich sources of Vitamin C. Vitamin C builds up protection against infection of every sort, including the common cold, and this same Vitamin C is essential for the building of sound teeth.

Vitamin D not only promotes quick healing of wounds, but is necessary for the absorption of calcium and phosphorus by the bones. In tomatoes and in milk, among other foods, this vitamin will be found. Furthermore in celery and in spinach, there is Vitamin E, which is important for its part in maintaining physical activity. This mysterious Vitamin E plays a definite role, too, in the endless struggle of women to keep the vitality and physical competence of youth.

The above summary of the part of vitamins, as present in raw fruits and vegetables, is brief and nonmedical. It is given merely to call attention to the importance of these vitamins in a diet called "Food for Beauty."

A detailed account of the nature of the minerals in

the foods used in this diet would necessarily become scientific and therefore be confusing to the layman. However, the importance of minerals in maintaining health cannot be overstressed, nor can the role raw fruits and vegetables play in supplying minerals be too loudly emphasized. From the viewpoint of the woman who seeks to retain her youth, we might pause to consider the signal importance of just one mineral element. Calcium is an outstanding need of the healthy human body. It plays an all-important part in growth and the continuance of health and vitality. Sherman reports on experiments in diets which will interest youth-seeking women (which really means every woman).*

"Hundreds of experimental animals have been studied throughout their lives to compare the effects of two diets which differ (among other things) in calcium content. On the diet richer in calcium the body increases its calcium content more rapidly during growth and also retains *the characteristics of youth* through a longer stretch of adult life before signs of old age appear. While the longer lease of healthier life conferred by the better of these two normal diets is not to be attributed solely to calcium, the more liberal calcium intake which expedites early development clearly appears to be advantageous throughout adult life as well."

Milk, used frequently in the *matière vivante* menus,

* *Food and Health* by Henry C. Sherman. By permission of The Macmillan Company, publishers.

is the primary source of calcium. The secondary sources of calcium are fruits and vegetables. Women who deliberately avoid milk in their reducing diets are starving themselves for calcium and at the same time acting under the delusion that skimmed milk is fattening.

You will find in the back of this book an entire section devoted to complete instructions on the preparation of special *matière vivante* meals for home use. These have been worked out with a full understanding of the average woman's domestic circumstances. Any woman can find the foods that have been selected in her local shops, no matter in what part of the country she lives, and can prepare them in her own kitchen in no more time than is needed for the usual home meals.

Should you try to make these luncheons as beautiful as possible? Is it really necessary? Yes, I think it is. I wish you would try to achieve a definite color and pattern harmony in the food you serve yourself. After all, you have started out on a pilgrimage. You are moving forward toward the secret hope of every normal woman—a spirited and internally clean body. From the state of tired nerves, intestinal sluggishness, a dry skin and vitamin-starved system, or from the equally unlovely state of overweight and consequent discouragement and lethargy, you now set forth along the highway up toward the achievement of complete and vital loveliness. *Certainly* there will be rough spots in the road, there will be discouragement waiting for you, the spirit will flag, for it is

only human to fail sometimes even in the most deep-
seated purpose. Beauty signposts along the way will be
like those shrines along the European roads which remind the traveler of the purpose of his pilgrimage through
life. Lovely colors before your eyes as you continue
this sunlight-nutrition diet and gorgeous patterns of raw
fruits and vegetables will frequently remind you of your
ultimate personal goal, so that when the flesh and spirit
tire, you will be encouraged and spurred onward by the
beautiful novelty of the food itself. It takes but little more
time to arrange these foods in eye-appealing patterns.
Certainly, all beauty-conscious women are aware of the
inspiration of gorgeous color. Why should you deny yourself the inspiration in the dancing colors of carefully
selected fruits and vegetables, particularly when it is so
easy to prepare them? You see why I urge you to come
as near as possible to artistic perfection in your food
arrangements. I know the value of these things. I have
seen the startling beauty of some of these meals. I know
what the sight of beauty has done to thousands of women.
It actually fires them with ambition. It in some subtle
way suggests the inner purpose of this entire system of
eating, and therefore holds them to their first resolve to
carry on until they, too, have been admitted to the ranks
of slender and vital women.

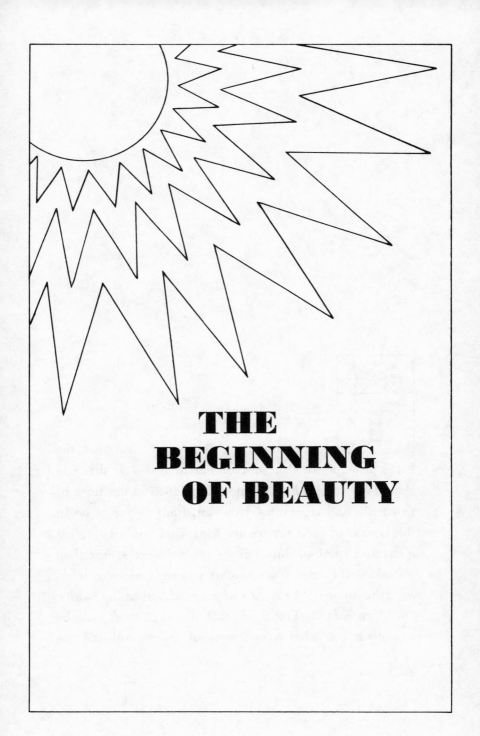

THE
BEGINNING
OF BEAUTY

I n the preceding chapter, I said that the basic principle of this sunlight-nutrition diet is that one should eat at least half of one's daily food in the form of raw fruits and vegetables. However, I advise you to begin this course of food for beauty with what might be called a curative routine. Only a few days, no more at first than a week, will be necessary to start you right in your determination to offset the results of years of bad eating habits.

You may at first think that this diet week will be strenuous. But what is one week of self-control and unusual food compared with years of overweight, physical discomfort, and a blemished skin? You were able to tolerate the unhappiness and nerve sag of these conditions for months, for years, maybe. Certainly you should welcome the hopeful thought of one week of a curative diet, which will be the dawn of a new health and the return of youth.

So please accept my advice and decide to adhere religiously to the curative diet for one week. After that you can follow the easier rule of 50 percent sunlight-nutrition food, with a 100 percent sunlight-nutrition diet day once a week, if possible. The more frequently you return to the 100 percent day, that much better will you be. Twice a year at least, you should take from one to three weeks of the curative diet.

Your beauty day begins at breakfast. You must rise from bed charged with hope. You have scientific reason for hope. The diet you have begun has cured thousands of men and women and has turned Zurich, Switzerland, where it originated, into the modern fountain of youth.

Stand before an open window and fill your lungs with fresh air. Do at least one stretching exercise—more if you can. Then comes your fragrant bath, a fresh rub down with eau de Cologne and you are ready for breakfast.

Remember, this is not a starvation diet. It is a healing diet. You have plenty of food to supply the body's demand for fuel, and you will have a sufficient variety of food to provide the minerals and vitamins necessary, as well as the minimum number of calories. The week ahead of you will be devoted to adjusting your metabolism. Your digestive organs and your circulation will be stimulated by the diet and the chemical powers of combustion throughout your entire system will be quickened. It is to be a week of clearance and revitalization.

For breakfast and supper the main dish will be Bircher-müesli. This is a combination of fruit, cereal, cream, and sweetening which can be varied in many ways, yet never ceases to be an ideal meal. The list of fresh fruits that you can select will be limited only by the season and the quality of your local markets.

APPLE BIRCHER-MÜESLI
(FOR ONE PERSON)

1 *level tablespoon finely rolled oats*
3 *tablespoons water*
  juice ½ lemon
1 *tablespoon or less of cream*
2 *apples*
  honey to taste

Soak rolled oats in the 3 tablespoons water for 12 hours. Then add lemon juice and cream. Mix thoroughly. Wash

38

apples but do not peel. Then grate the apples into the oat mixture, and stir well. Serve at once.

The entire apple is grated into the mixture, including skin, core, and pips. By using the entire apple you greatly increase the amount of valuable minerals in the müesli. Soda, magnesia, oxide of iron, sulphuric acid, and silicic acid are contained in the skin, core, and seeds. The increase in these nutritive minerals means a quicker improvement in body tone. The silicic acid content of the müesli is of great importance in the health of the eyes, skin, and hair.

In preparing this dish for yourself, do not increase the proportion of oats in the mistaken belief that you need more nourishment. The fruit is the main factor in the value of this dish. What few calories that are needed are supplied by the oats, cream, and small amount of honey, a total of approximately 210 calories. That's plenty for you at this time. The fruit is not only curative in its action, but also has nutritive value. It will all be used up in the digestive tract, provided it is finely grated.

If the müesli seems too scant a dish, add a few chopped nut meats to it. Stir in well at the last moment. The consistency of nuts will increase the pleasure of eating this Swiss dish and of course will also add protein.

Before the müesli, eat an orange or half a grapefruit. Use the juice if you prefer. But do not strain. The cellulose of unstrained juice is valuable in the regulation of the intestinal tract.

What, a cold breakfast! The idea makes you shudder! It really shouldn't. In Zurich, where the winters are severe, they eat this breakfast regularly. The body has its own warming equipment. If you eat and drink this food slowly, a little at a time, the esophagus will warm it properly and it will reach the stomach at the correct temperature. Every time you put the body to work as it was designed to work, you increase its health and improve its tone. The average diet of hot soft cooked food, with its spices and condiments, does not require the digestive organs to function as they are intended to function. Consequently, the natural sense of taste, the thermostatic system and the muscles of the digestive tract all get lazy.

However, despite all that has just been said, if you cannot at once accustom yourself to cold food, then warm the müesli slightly. You may even dilute your fruit juice with hot water. But try not to, or at least resolve to abandon this practice as soon as you possibly can.

During your week of curative diet which begins your Food for Beauty way of eating, it is wise to vary the fruit used in the müesli. Only the fruit is varied; the proportion of cereal and cream remains the same.

Strawberries, raspberries, blackberries, blueberries, currants, or gooseberries can make delightful changes in the berry müesli. For fruit müesli, you have fresh apricots, peaches, plums, cherries, nectarines, on through the list. Bananas make an economical dish too, especially for a build-up diet.

To make the berry müesli, use 5¼ oz. mashed berry pulp. Wash the berries carefully, drain and then either mash or put through grinder. Use all the berries, including the seeds. Follow instructions for making apple müesli, substituting the berry pulp for the grated apples.

To make the fresh fruit müesli, use 5½ oz. of prepared fruit. Wash the fruit carefully, remove pits but not the skin. Then put fruit through the grinder or else chop fine. Then use in place of the grated apple in the standard müesli recipe.

For banana müesli, remove skin, put fruit through grinder or else mash, and stir at once into prepared oats to prevent discoloration. This is excellent for children and underweight persons.

If no fresh fruits are available, then dried fruits, such as prunes, apples, apricots, and peaches can be used in Bircher-müesli.

Wash the dried fruit first in hot water. Then soak in cold water for 24 hours. Even after this soaking, the fruit will need very careful mastication to enable the digestive organs to utilize the material. Put the soaked dried fruit through the grinder, using the finest blade.

To make dried fruit müesli, use 3½ oz. of the prepared fruit instead of the 5¼ oz. of the fresh fruit. Then follow the standard recipe for Bircher-müesli.

So much for breakfast during your curative week. It

41

will be Bircher-müesli after orange or grapefruit or other fruit. Nothing else. It should be served at room temperature, but if you feel you are not yet ready to begin your day without something hot, then warm this curative and energizing food slightly. The main thing is to get started along the path of streamlined and vibrant health.

Bircher-müesli will appear again at supper during your diet week. The fruits can be different if you like.

Later on, when you reduce the proportion of raw fruits and vegetables in your sunlight-nutrition diet, you can use Bircher-müesli as the main breakfast dish. But serve with it whole-wheat bread, a glass of milk, or a cup of herbal tea. The valuable contents of müesli, vitamins and minerals in organic combinations as well as its natural flavors, make it a dish of great importance. The sooner you accustom yourself to making and using it, the better for your health and appearance.

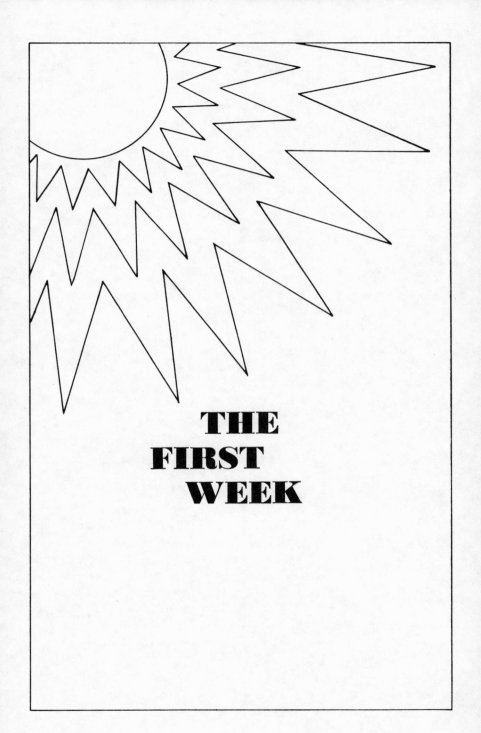

THE
FIRST
WEEK

You are starting your first week of Food for Beauty. You will lose from two to three pounds safely while you also recondition your entire system. Your beauty diet day has just begun. You have had breakfast and know that Bircher-müesli will reappear at supper. But what will there be for the midday meal? Even women seeking lovelier skins and more vital health are human, and "What will there be for dinner?" is a very human question.

Your main meal will consist of fruits and vegetables,

fresh and unspoiled by the process of cooking. They will be delicious with the flavors brought to them by the sun and gay to look at in their natural colors. Yes, the meal will consist of raw fruits and vegetables as they come from the sun-warmed orchards and gardens. A few nuts and a little cream cheese with garden herbs will supply the protein necessary for the complete combustion of the other food.

Perhaps the novelty of the idea of rawness will cause you to forget what was said earlier. Your digestive system can take care of raw foods, despite your belief to the contrary. When Professor C. C. Furnas of Yale University discussed this sunlight-nutrition diet of raw fruits and vegetables in the Zurich Room, he was enthusiastic. He referred me to certain passages of *Man, Bread and Destiny* which he wrote in collaboration with S. M. Furnas, formerly instructor in Nutrition at the University of Minnesota. If you are puzzled over what raw food will do to you, and you need further reassurance, then read these lines from *Man, Bread and Destiny.**

"Almost everyone knows that cooking increases digestibility but almost everyone is wrong about that," Professor Furnas states. "With some exceptions cooking does not increase the ultimate assimilability of foods and, particularly if overdone, or at too high a temperature, often has the reverse effect. *Rats* almost always show

* Quoted through the courtesy of Reynal & Hitchcock.

46

greater growth and greater intestinal happiness if fed on raw rather than cooked foods."

Professor Furnas makes another statement which is particularly enlightening for women on this diet. He writes, "Cooking has no effect on the ultimate assimilation—it merely shortens the time in which it is accomplished."

Raw foods, as indicated by the above statements, are assimilated as thoroughly as cooked foods. You will be surprised, as so many thousands of other women have been, at the hunger-satisfying quality of a dinner of raw fruits and vegetables. You will go for several hours without desire for more food, perfectly well-nourished and without that heavy feeling which so often follows the family main meal. That is because the raw foods are relatively not so quickly assimilated, though of course their ultimate assimilation is complete.

The sunlight main meal you will serve your mineral and vitamin hungry body should be comprised of three types of vegetables. And, of course, some fruit. They may be selected according to your personal preference, though within a reasonably short time you will discover undreamed of flavors in almost all raw vegetables.

Roughly, though not completely, you can classify the vegetables into these three groups for convenience:

1. FRUIT OF THE PLANT: tomatoes, cucumbers, squash, pumpkin, melons, etc.

2. LEAF OF THE PLANT: lettuce, endive, dandelion greens, spinach, cresses, cabbage, Brussels sprouts, chicory, fennell, and aromatic leaves, such as chives, parsley, chervil, tarragon, etc.

3. ROOT OF THE PLANT: carrots, radishes, beets, onions, leeks, kohlrabi, shallots, potatoes, etc.

The leguminous plants—peas and beans—must be included in your vegetables. They are important sources of vegetable protein.

Make your first vegetable dish simple. Later on you can experiment and greatly increase the variety and pleasing combinations. The following is given as an example. In a later chapter you will find more recipes for these *matière vivante* meals.

FOOD FOR BEAUTY PLATE
(FOR ONE PERSON)

4 *firm lettuce leaves*
1 *carrot*
3 *radishes*
½ *small leek*
2 *young spinach leaves*
1 *small tomato*
1 *tablespoon shelled green peas*

Wash the vegetables carefully. Shred the carrot and the leek. Slice the radishes into thin discs with a sharp knife. Chop the spinach leaves and green peas separately. Cut the unpeeled tomato into small pieces.

In the center of the plate, place one lettuce leaf and in it lay the cut up tomato. Arrange the three remaining lettuce cups about the plate, forming an attractive arrangement. Now fill each of these—3 cups with the prepared vegetables in whatever combinations seem most pleasing to you.

Sprinkle a little lemon juice over the vegetables and a few drops of olive oil. Do not use any salt, if possible, or other seasoning. Chop a few walnuts and use them as extra flavoring. You will discover that nuts give delightful taste to your food.

Serve immediately. This type of food cannot be prepared long in advance. Freshness and crispness are important.

That is the main dish of the main meal of the day. You begin with a 5 oz. glass of fresh fruit juice or fresh vegetable juice, or with a combination of vegetable and fruit juices.

Your dessert can be an apple, an orange, a plum, or any other fruit you enjoy. It must of course be eaten without sugar or cream or salt.

On the first day of your week of curative diet, your total food intake will contain about 500 calories. That is a low but not a starvation caloric diet. It differs from many reducing diets in this way—it contains all the elements needed by the body, including minerals, vitamins, and proteins. It will rest the digestive tract and not harm it. And you will not have any sense of being starved.

Your eating time table for the curative-reducing week will be as follows. On the first day, breakfast consists of Bircher-müesli, a slice of whole wheat bread, and one serving of butter. You may have fruit juice, hot herbal tea, or lemon juice. In any of these beverages on the first day you may take one lump of sugar.

The main meal will begin with a 5 oz. glass of fresh fruit or vegetable juice, or with a combination of fruit and vegetable juices. These juices must always be sipped very slowly. That is very important to remember. Then comes the main dish, consisting of at least three raw vegetables, served as described a few paragraphs back. With this *matière vivante* plate, you may have one slice of whole wheat bread and one serving of butter. Dessert will be fresh fruit served plain.

For supper, you may have Bircher-müesli, fruit or vegetable juice, or whole fruit, and a 5 oz. glass of skimmed milk. If you prefer, you may use different fruits from those used for breakfast.

On the second day of your curative-reducing week, you serve the same principal foods. But several accessory foods must be left out. At breakfast, leave out the whole wheat bread and butter, and also the one lump of sugar with your beverage.

For luncheon on the second day, leave out the whole wheat bread and butter, and for supper, serve only raw fruit and Bircher-müesli.

On the third day, as well as the fifth and seventh day of this first week, repeat the first day's schedule of eating. On the fourth and sixth days, repeat the second day's schedule.

Do not drink water with these meals. You will not need it. Vegetables and fruits are more than 75 percent liquid and will therefore supply your tissues with all the liquid necessary. Furthermore, you are introducing large quantities of vegetable cellulose into your digestive tract. Only a little of this will be absorbed, the rest will have a tonic effect on the intestinal tract. However, if you drink excessive quantities of water while eating raw fruits and vegetables, the water will act on the cellulose, causing the cellulose to increase in bulk. Too much cellulose may irritate a sensitive intestinal tract. But the amounts of liquid contained in the vegetables given for these curative days will be in proper proportion to other cellulose content.

CURATIVE DIET

1st Day, 3rd Day, 5th Day, 7th Day

BREAKFAST

orange or ½ grapefruit
Müesli
1 slice whole wheat toast
herbal tea
1 lump sugar

MAIN MEAL

5 oz. fruit or vegetable juice
Food for Beauty plate
1 slice whole wheat bread
1 serving butter
raw fruit

SUPPER

fruit juice or fruit
Müesli
5 oz. skim milk

CURATIVE DIET

2nd Day, 4th Day, 6th Day

BREAKFAST

orange or ½ grapefruit
Müesli
herbal tea

MAIN MEAL

5 oz. fruit or vegetable juice
Food for Beauty plate
(without peas or beans)
raw fruit

SUPPER

raw fresh fruit
Müesli

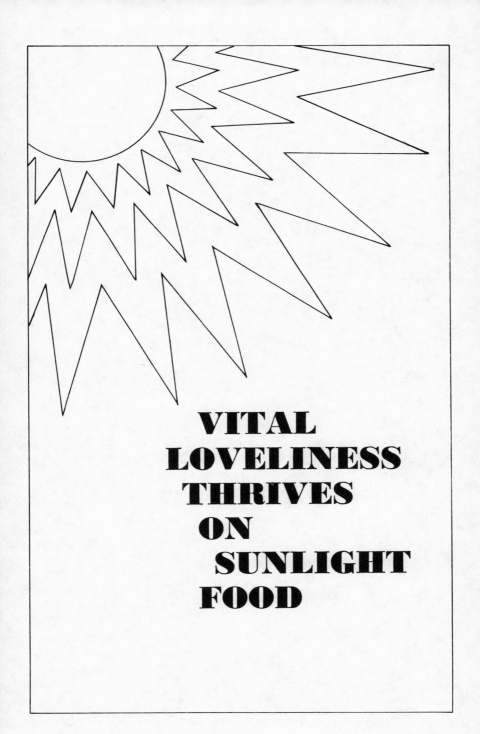

**VITAL
LOVELINESS
THRIVES
ON
SUNLIGHT
FOOD**

Y ou have completed your curative-reducing week of diet. Your system has been revitalized and you are ready now to continue "Food for Beauty" as a new way of eating. Life offers you hope, and radiant youthfulness promises to become far more lasting than you had even dared hope.

How long should you continue to nourish your body and spirits on Food for Beauty? I hope you will continue to eat this way as long as you live. This remarkable system of nutrition is not only for overweight women and or for women who sag in muscle and in vitality because of bad eating habits and vitamin starving. Certainly for such women it is the great answer and will lead them back to normal slenderness and a renaissance of vitality.

Later in this book, I describe the particular diets to be followed for varying degrees of overweight and other abnormal conditions. But in this chapter, I appeal to the intelligence of normal women who now realize that the continuance of their abundant health can be insured by faithful and permanent adherence to this diet.

You are youthful, in normal health, buoyant, and lovely. You want to stay that way. Then resolve to protect your state of beauty with sunlight foods. But carry your resolution to its logical conclusions. Include your husband, your children and other members of your household in the resolution. In other words, reorganize your family's eating habits. Greater health, sturdiness, and happiness for your household will reward your efforts.

A moderately active person of normal weight needs about 2,200 to 2,500 calories a day to maintain his energy. However, one needs many other food elements than calories. The daily food allowance must be rich in mineral elements and should be more than adequate in all the vitamins.

This maintenance diet for healthy people who want to stay healthy must be at least half raw fruits and vegetables. It is, however, not a vegetarian diet. It allows for the use of meat and fish, but only when roasted, boiled, or broiled—never fried. It includes a moderate amount of starches and also permits the use of sugar in limited and reasonable amounts. Most of the sweet-tooth requirements are met with the fresh fruits.

You may not be too pleased at first at giving up your puddings, pies, and pastries. But you have decided to eat for health and internal happiness, remember. Bad eating habits are to be overcome. And one of the worst eating habits in America is the abnormal consumption of sugar.

Henry C. Sherman, Mitchell Professor of Chemistry, Columbia University, and one of the greatest recognized living authorities on food and diet, points this out in his standard book, *Food and Health*.* He writes as follows: "With the exception of molasses, sorghum, and sugar cane syrup, all of which retain a significant proportion of the mineral elements of the plant juices, sugars and syrups make their sole contribution to the diet through their carbohydrate content.

"It is estimated that in the United States today, about one-fourth of the energy requirement is got through eating sugar in its various forms. With this large proportion of the total energy intake in the form of such a one-sided food, it follows that the intake of protein, phosphorous, calcium, iron, and vitamins is on the whole proportionately diminished. Investigations of recent years indicate strongly this trend is contrary to good nutritional

* *Food and Health* by Henry C. Sherman. By permission of The Macmillan Company, publishers.

practices and that the American people would benefit if sugar consumption were reduced and the needed energy obtained from the consumption of other food material. Probably the desire for sweet-eating foods is best satisfied by the eating of fruits."

In the diet menus for the daily food allowance required for the moderately active man or woman, provision is made for the 2,200 to 2,500 calories needed and given at the end of this chapter for a super-abundance of vitamins and minerals. These daily menus are presented merely as guides to show you how to include the minimum 50 percent essential amount of raw fruits and vegetables in the adaptation for American homes of the Bircher-Benner sunlight-nutrition diet. There are four daily menus given for guides, and each one takes into consideration the vegetables and fruits generally available during the seasons of fall, winter, spring, and summer. You will soon learn how to make your own daily menus from these sample seasonal menus. The markets will suggest endless variations of fruits and vegetables from which you can create health bringing meals for every day in the year.

Once again, let me state the basic principle—at least half of the food allowance per person per day must be in the form of raw fruits and vegetables.

One of the most delightful and also nutritionally correct ways of serving the required quota of raw fruits and vegetables in the daily menu is to use the full *matière vivante* luncheon made famous in the Zurich Room. In a subsequent chapter, the *matière vivante* plates, which are the basis of the Zurich Room luncheons, are given in complete detail. The recipes will enable you to serve in your own home the now famous crystal plates on which some of the most beautiful and fashionable women in the world maintained the health that underlies their beauty.

In the same chapter, there are recipes for simplified domestic versions of these same famous dishes. They are for women who cannot spend so much time on preparation of these foods, yet wish to follow the diets regularly.

When should these Zurich Room meals be served in your home? You will have to answer that question yourself. The answer will depend entirely on your family's activities. If all the family meets for a midday meal, then use the Zurich Room luncheon at that time.

However, if your husband does not return until evening, and you have convinced him that this maintenance diet is the answer to his secret fears that the years are beginning to tell on his face and formerly athletic figure, you will have to plan differently. Serve this Zurich Room meal once or twice a week for dinner. The rest of the week serve it at midday, but remind your husband that for his luncheon he must select foods from the restaurant menu which will not lower his average of 50 percent raw fruits and vegetables as a daily requirement.

Now let us study this Zurich Room meal in detail.

It contains about 300 calories, plus even more than

the required amounts of minerals and vitamins. It consists of 5 oz. of fresh vegetable or fruit juice, an assortment of raw fruits and vegetables all finely shredded, chopped, or cut, a few chopped nuts or a little herbal cream cheese. For dessert, an apple, an orange, a pear, grapes, or any other fruit desired.

This same meal belongs in the maintenance diet. With it are served some form of zwieback, rusk, or whole wheat bread and one helping of butter.

After the raw fruit and vegetable plate, serve a cup of clear, unsalted herbal bouillon. To make this very palatable bouillon, place several greens in an enamel pot. Use the trimmed off parts of celery, lettuce, carrots, leeks—use any green or vegetable at hand, add a very little cold water. Bring slowly to simmer, then simmer gently for about 20 minutes. The rule can be simplified as follows: Use a large quantity of greens and vegetables, very little water, simmer for 20 minutes, strain, and serve hot. Do not use salt or any other seasoning. The vegetables are full of delicious flavors themselves.

The cup of hot bouillon is served after the raw vegetable plate, never before it. It is an added source of liquid, minerals, and vitamins, and will add a little diversion to this diet meal.

The meal with the foods just described will contain approximately 300 calories.

Remember, the special diet we are now studying is a maintenance diet, not a slenderizing one. Its purpose is to build and maintain vigorous health and it can be used regularly all year in the home for all members of your family. It is also the perfect way to teach yourself and your growing family scientifically correct eating habits.

The daily amounts of food provided by the above menus will maintain the averagely active man or woman in optimal health. For children and adolescents, who require more food because their bodies are going through the building process, from a pint and a half to one quart of milk a day must be added.

Additional milk and baked potatoes with or without the skins may be desirable for some children, a fact to be determined by your physician.

As to the use of tea and coffee in the maintenance diet for normal people, more will be said later on. For the present, the use is permitted, if reluctantly.

To some, these maintenance diets will seem very generous. To others, they will look like the first steps toward starvation. What they really are, however, is the fundamental requirements in all the food elements to keep a normal body healthy and toned up to its best possible condition.

The inclusion of raw fruits and vegetables to a proportion of 50 percent or more is the outstanding feature. The elimination from the daily diet of excess amounts of sugar is another.

For heavy eaters, for women who weigh far in excess

of their height and age standards, this maintenance diet will become a reducing diet insofar as it will bring down their excess weight—slowly but permanently.

There are many women who wish to follow this maintenance diet for their health and figure, although they do not keep house. Those who must eat luncheon and dinner in restaurants and yet adhere to the two basic rules of their maintenance diet—(1) at least 50 percent of the daily food in the form of raw fruits and vegetables (2) a maximum of 2,500 calories a day—will have to study each menu carefully and select first from fruit juices, fruit cups, fruit and vegetable salads. When their 50 percent quota has been met, they can select the remainder of the meal from cooked items on the menu.

Sample menus for the maintenance diet of 2,500 calories, in which 50 percent of the food is in the form of raw fruits and vegetables.

One full day menu is given for each of the four seasons of the year. Use these sample menus to help you plan your Food for Beauty meals every day in the year.

FALL

BREAKFAST

glass grapefruit juice

boiled egg   4 thin strips bacon

2 slices whole wheat toast   butter

tea or coffee or lemon and hot water

(cream and 1 teaspoon sugar)

10 A.M.   1 glass milk

LUNCHEON

fruit or vegetable juice

3 to 6 raw vegetables

nuts, French dressing—herbal cream cheese ball

zwieback, rusk, or whole wheat bread   butter

herbal bouillon

fruit

DINNER

large mixed raw vegetable salad   French dressing

clear green pea soup

broiled steak

baked Hubbard squash   buttered string beans

whole wheat bread   butter

sliced bananas with lemon juice

demitasse

BEDTIME   glass of fruit juice

This day's menu contains about 2,200 calories. For growing children and adolescents, add at least 3 more glasses of milk and a baked potato.

WINTER

BREAKFAST

5 oz. orange juice

Bircher-müesli

2 slices whole wheat toast   butter

tea or coffee, lemon juice and hot water

(cream and 1 teaspoon sugar)

10 A.M.   1 glass vegetable juice

LUNCHEON

fruit or vegetable juice

6 fresh raw fruits and vegetables   French dressing

zwieback, rusk, or whole wheat bread

nuts   cream cheese ball

herbal bouillon

fruit

DINNER

salad of lettuce, chicory, and sliced tomato

French dressing

1 cup clear vegetable broth

1 serving roast beef

1 medium browned potato

1 serving broccoli with melted butter

1 slice whole wheat bread   butter

½ grapefruit with 1 teaspoon raw cane sugar

demitasse

BEDTIME   1 glass orange and lemon juice

For growing children and adolescents, follow instructions for
increasing calories for fall diet.

SPRING

BREAKFAST

1 large serving strawberries
cream   raw cane sugar
1 slice broiled ham   1 poached egg
2 slices whole wheat toast   butter
tea or coffee, lemon juice and hot water
(cream and 1 teaspoon sugar)

10 A.M.   *5 oz. fresh tomato and fresh celery juice*

LUNCHEON

fruit or vegetable juice
3 to 6 raw vegetables and fruits   French dressing
nuts   cottage cheese
zwieback, rusk, or whole wheat bread   butter
spring greens bouillon
fruit

DINNER

mixed spring greens salad   (cresses, lettuce,
radishes, cucumber, tomato, young dandelion greens)
mushroom bouillon
½ broiled chicken
6 stalks fresh asparagus   drawn butter
whole wheat bread   carrots in cream
sliced orange with grated fresh coconut
demitasse

BEDTIME   *glass of orange juice*

For growing children and adolescents, include at least 3 glasses
of milk and one serving of potato.

SUMMER

BREAKFAST

½ cantaloupe
Bircher-müesli
2 slices raisin toast   butter
coffee or tea, lemon juice and hot water
(cream and 1 teaspoon sugar)

10 A.M.   *5 oz. fresh green vegetable juice*

LUNCHEON

fruit or vegetable juice
3 to 6 raw spring vegetables   French dressing
nuts, herbal cream cheese ball
zwieback, rusk or whole wheat bread   butter
lima bean bouillon
fruit

DINNER

fresh fruit salad   (fresh pineapple,
pear, orange, lettuce and French dressing)
garden bouillon
2 broiled lamb chops
parsley potato balls   new peas
whole wheat bread   butter
fresh raspberries
whipped cream   powdered sugar
demitasse

BEDTIME   *5 oz. blueberry and lemon juice*

For growing children and adolescents, add at least 3 glasses of whole milk daily.

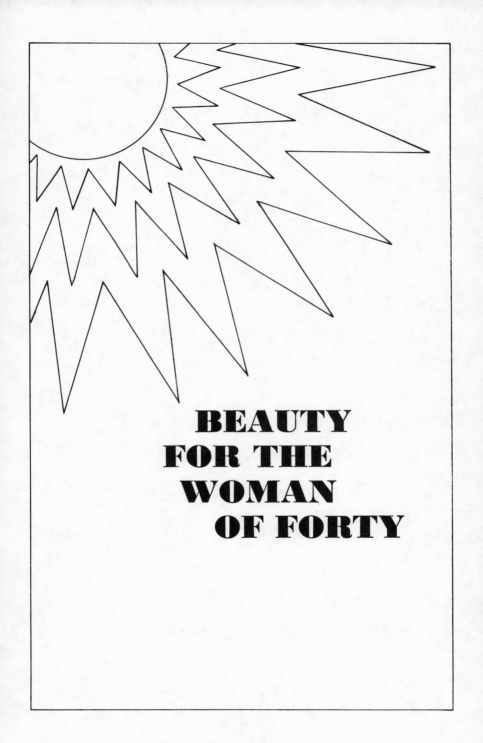

BEAUTY
FOR THE
WOMAN
OF FORTY

You are a woman of forty. You want to look younger and to streamline your figure. What should you do?

You should do many things. But we are talking about diet now, so let's discuss the food required to bring back youthfulness in looks, figure, and spirits.

Should you go on a starvation diet in order to keep slim? No—definitely no. The rule for a woman of forty is the rule of perfect health. And that rule of perfect health is the same as the rule for good looks. In other words, Food for Beauty is basically food for health.

71

The excess poundage that may spoil the figure when a woman approaches the interesting age has nothing to do with years. Extra weight is not necessarily a concomitant of years. It is rather the result of an appetite that is more eager than the needs of the body. Every ounce of food taken into the body which is not consumed as fuel turns into fat. But note this point—every ounce of food which the body needs does not turn into fat.

In early life, the body is in the process of being built. The processes of growth demand larger quantities of food, naturally. But by the age of thirty, these constructive needs decrease because the physical structure has been about completed. From then on, although, of course, the body must be maintained in perfect condition, extra material for building is no longer needed. From thirty on, food should be eaten only for maintenance.

Between thirty and forty, the average modern American woman is interested in sports. She is active, alert, a spirited being. Although her body does not need extra food for building purposes, it does need fuel for her physical activities. Her diet, consequently, must be up to the energy needs of her activities. Although she will not require as many calories as she did when she was still under thirty, she will require a reasonably large supply of fuel food, around 2,500 calories a day.

However, if the woman around thirty leads a sedentary life, either in an office where she gets little or no exercise, or else in an environment of ease and inactivity, wherein automobiles and yachts relieve her of the need to use her muscles, her diet should be reduced accordingly in excess calories. Otherwise, she will find to her dismay that she is spreading around the hips. Yes, that is a thing most ardently to be avoided in the name of beauty—and in the name of vital health.

When she reaches forty, the average woman does not exercise as much as her younger sister. But some regular exercise, of course, in less strenuous form, must be part of her daily routine for beauty. Daily streamlining exercise is as important as care of her skin with wisely chosen creams and lotions.

It must be apparent that as her fuel-consuming exercises grow less, the woman of forty will need fewer calories in her diet. And as the building processes of her body no longer go on, she must deny herself food that was needed during the building stage. In other words, the woman of forty who seeks a graceful figure must realize that she must not continue eating as much food as she did during her twenties and thirties.

Nature, however, has her little joke, and plays it too often at the cost of a woman's youthful appearance. Despite the decreasing need for fuel foods, and despite the tendency to take less and less strenuous part in tennis, golf, swimming and riding, the human appetite goes right on being as active as it was in girlhood. As a result, a woman without self-restraint will eat herself into excess weight and unbecoming bulk, believing she must keep up her strength.

Every calorie of food eaten, which is not required

by the normally functioning body, turns into dreaded fat. However, and fortunately, calories are far from being the only food elements required to keep the body in vital health. A clear skin, glistening hair, and an active digestive system demand their supply of the regulating minerals and vitamins. These, as we have seen, are bountifully supplied by vegetables and fruit.

Intestinal health is perhaps the greatest need of the woman of forty who cherishes her appearance. The beauty of her face and the suppleness of her body depend to an amazing extent on the healthy condition of her intestinal system. In other words, constipation is the arch enemy of beauty in women. Constipation in most cases is nothing more than the result of bad eating habits.

Rather than protest myself against the evil habit so many otherwise modern and progressive women have of using cathartics and strong intestinal abrasives to a dangerous excess, I shall quote the words of Dr. Henry C. Sherman, again referring to his *Food and Health*.*

"Fruits and many vegetables also have an important relation to the maintenance of good conditions in the intestines. This is largely because of the bulk which they impart to the residues, thus giving the muscular mechanism of the intestine a chance to be effective in keeping the residual mass moving and ensuring its elimination without undue delay, the fiber of these foods also serving to

* *Food and Health* by Henry C. Sherman. By permission of The Macmillan Company, publishers.

give the digestive apparatus 'its daily scrubbing.' This effect is, of course, shared by the grain products which have not been too highly refined. Bran particles may easily be more laxative, but the softer cellulose of *fruits and tender vegetables* may be very important to intestinal hygiene in those cases in which an equal volume of bran residue would be too harsh.

"Most fruits and vegetables have also another valuable property, especially when eaten raw, in that the chewing of their fiber in the presence of the mild acids which the fruits and vegetables naturally contain is extremely effective in preventing the retention of pasty particles or mucus upon the teeth, while the acid also stimulates the flow of the saliva and the gastric juice. Thus the digestive process is helped and the mouth is left in the best possible condition. Hence the great wholesomeness of raw fruit or fruit salad as a dessert, or of the eating of some celery or raw apple at the very end of (or directly after) a meal. Either the whole, or a half, or a quarter of a raw apple may be taken as preferred; best eaten with the skin, having been well washed before quartering —any surface not effectively reached in washing being rejected with the core."

A diet of raw fruits and vegetables, in conjunction with restricted amounts of other foods, takes on added importance for the woman of forty who seeks to maintain both her health and her figure. It will supply bulk, which is needed to keep her intestinal mechanism in effective condition. Furthermore, and I believe this point is highly important to the hungry forties, raw fruits and vegetables with their wealth of pleasing flavors and variety of consistencies, as well as their beautiful colors and appeal to the appetite through the eye, give the woman who must not overeat the impression that she is eating a great deal. A handsomely arranged luncheon of several raw fruits and vegetables presents a large and appetizing appearance, despite its welcome deficiency in excess calories.

Just how much should you eat each day now that you have achieved the interesting and significant age of forty? That question cannot be answered without some consideration of your activities, your height, and your weight. There are, especially in the United States, a great number of women whose activities in business and social life make the average teen-age girl seem tired and old. However, by and large, the great majority of women begin to be less active physically at this time. For them the limited but by no means insufficient diet given below will supply them with all the calories they need, and more than supply them with those energizing and esprit maintaining vitamins and minerals.

This diet contains about 1,200 calories a day, all the heat-giving units required by a body that has been structurally completed and that is not very active in a physical way. For anyone of any age, who is very much overweight and who is tall, this same diet will do wonders in taking off those ugly pounds that destroy appearance and make the spirit sluggish.

Once again I call your attention to the basic rule of Food for Beauty. Of all the food you eat during the day, at least one half of it must be raw fruits and vegetables. In the following Food for Beauty menus, that rule is followed. To make it easier for you to follow this diet in your own home, four sets of sample menus are given, each one using fruits and vegetables generally available in the markets during the four seasons of the year.

FALL

—1200 calories

BREAKFAST

5 oz. glass orange juice
2 strips crisp bacon
1 slice melba toast   margarine
coffee without cream or sugar

10 A.M.   *5 oz. tomato juice*

LUNCHEON

chicken and raw vegetable salad
reducing mayonnaise*
2 slices melba toast
fresh fruit cup
coffee or tea—without cream or sugar

4 P.M.   *5 oz. grapefruit juice*

DINNER

fruit juice
small lettuce salad with raw carrot and
green peppers, julienne
reducing dressing**
broiled lean beefsteak   baked acorn squash
fresh pear with cream cheese
black coffee

BEDTIME   *1 large glass buttermilk*

* See recipe, pp. 111–12.
** See recipe, pp. 110–11.

WINTER

—1200 calories

BREAKFAST

½ grapefruit
Bircher-müesli
coffee or tea without cream or sugar

10 A.M.   5 oz. fresh vegetable juice

LUNCHEON

pineapple, cabbage, and tomato salad
reducing dressing
2 slices melba toast   1 unpeeled apple
tea or skim milk

4 P.M.   5 oz. glass skim milk
or buttermilk

DINNER

fruit juice
endive with grated raw celery, and chopped raw spinach
reducing dressing
clear vegetable bouillon
1 serving roast turkey
cranberry sauce sweetened with sugar substitute
Brussels sprouts
sliced orange with grated fresh coconut
black coffee

BEDTIME   5 oz. fruit juice

SPRING

—1200 calories

BREAKFAST

5 oz. orange juice
2 slices melba toast
margarine
coffee without cream or sugar

10 A.M.   *small glass fruit juice*
with egg white beaten into it

LUNCHEON

fresh fruit salad
reducing dressing
2 slices dry toast
tea or coffee without cream or sugar

4 P.M.   *5 oz. vegetable juice*

DINNER

fruit juice
small mixed green salad   reducing dressing
hot essence of green peas
roast leg of lamb
string beans   new carrots
honeydew melon

BEDTIME   *5 oz. skim milk*

SUMMER

—1200 calories

BREAKFAST

blueberries with whole milk
2 slices melba toast   margarine
coffee without cream or sugar

10 A.M.   *small glass fruit juice or*
piece of whole fruit

LUNCHEON

5 oz. fruit juice
large raw vegetable salad   reducing dressing
herbal cream cheese
2 slices melba toast
coffee or tea without cream or sugar

4 P.M.   *5 oz. tomato juice*

DINNER

hearts of lettuce, quartered, unpeeled
tomatoes, shredded raw carrot and celery
reducing dressing
hot essence of green beans
2 slices roast chicken
new peas   1 small ear corn
1 fresh pear
coffee or tea without cream or sugar

BEDTIME   *glass buttermilk or fruit juice*

Perhaps the woman of forty who seeks to maintain the spirit and vitality of her younger days will want still another diet to vary the routine of her Food for Beauty. The one that follows will interest her also. It was prepared by my personal physician, a man noted in the East for his success in treating women who suffer from loss of spirit and enthusiasm for life. Many times, of course, there is a psychological basis for their sag. But more often, he tells me, incorrect eating habits and lack of any intelligent exercise are the cause of what his patients incorrectly believe to be signs of approaching age.

The diet he recommends is simple and adequate. For the overweight woman, it will serve as a moderate reducing diet. For the woman whose weight is right for her height-age, this is an excellent maintenance diet.

FIRST DAY

BREAKFAST

½ *grapefruit*
1 cup of black coffee (no sugar)

LUNCHEON

½ *grapefruit*
1 egg
1 slice of melba toast

DINNER

2 eggs
1 tomato
½ *head of lettuce*
grapefruit
tea (no sugar or cream)

SECOND DAY

BREAKFAST

½ grapefruit
1 cup of black coffee (no sugar)

LUNCHEON

1 orange
1 egg
½ slice of melba toast

DINNER

broiled steak
½ head of lettuce
1 tomato
½ grapefruit

THIRD DAY

BREAKFAST

½ *grapefruit*
1 cup of black coffee (no sugar)

LUNCHEON

½ *grapefruit*
1 egg
½ *head of lettuce*
tea

DINNER

½ *grapefruit*
3 radishes
½ *head of lettuce*
tea or black coffee

FOURTH DAY

BREAKFAST

½ grapefruit
1 cup of black coffee (no sugar)

LUNCHEON

½ grapefruit
1 oz. favorite cheese
1 tomato
1 slice of melba toast
tea

DINNER

½ grapefruit
broiled steak
watercress or lettuce

FIFTH DAY

BREAKFAST

½ grapefruit
1 cup of black coffee (no sugar)

LUNCHEON

1 orange
1 lamb chop
½ head of lettuce
tea

DINNER

½ grapefruit
2 eggs
lettuce and tomato
tea

SIXTH DAY

BREAKFAST

½ *grapefruit*
1 cup of black coffee (no sugar)

LUNCHEON

1 orange
tea

DINNER

1 poached egg
1 slice of melba toast
1 orange
tea

SEVENTH DAY

BREAKFAST

½ *grapefruit*
1 cup of black coffee (no sugar)

LUNCHEON

½ *grapefruit*
2 eggs
lettuce and tomato
tea

DINNER

2 lamb chops
lettuce and tomato
tea or demitasse

AVOID ALL SWEETS, STARCHES, SUGAR, AND CREAM.

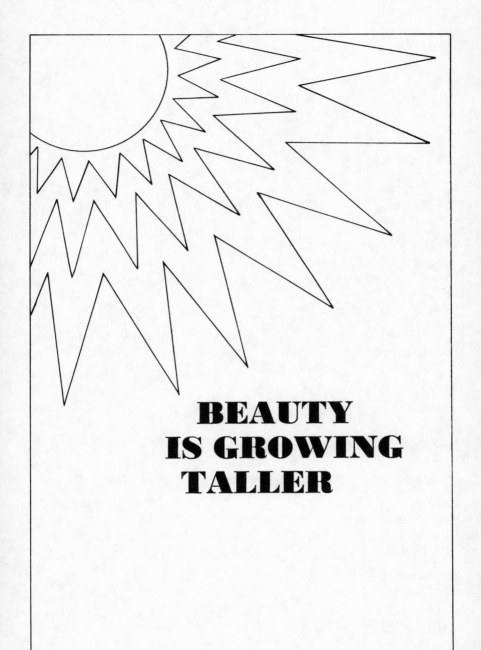

**BEAUTY
IS GROWING
TALLER**

It is true that the young woman of today tends to be far taller than her mother and her grandmother. Scientists explain the increase in height of our younger generation to the improvement in the American diet. Our children have been nourished up into vigorous and slender young manhood and young womanhood on a diet in which fruits, vegetables, and milk played a vital part. They are a handsome and agile breed and should stand as daily reminders of the need of vitamins and minerals for the healthy body.

When a tall person neglects her diet and puts on unwanted pounds above the hips, it is not very difficult to reduce her back to her normal slenderness. I have often found that the tall woman who weighs more than she should is quicker to realize the need of saner diet and a little more inclined to follow the routine of raw fruits and vegetables. But the short woman, for whom every excess pound appears to take on the weight of two, seems to find dieting and exercising extremely difficult. There is no royal road to streamlined beauty, alas, and the short heavy woman, no matter what age, should banish her lethargy, take hope, and resolve to achieve the grace and petite figure which lies hidden beneath those layers of fat. Candies, pudding, gravies, and alcohol are arch enemies to her youthful beauty. But the fresh fruits and vegetables from lovely gardens and shaded orchards are her vitalizing friends. Many times I have seen listless and dumpy short women turn into vivacious and willowy creatures after faithful months on the sunlight-nutrition diet. I know that you, too, despite whatever unkind truths your bathroom scales tell you and despite your fears that your will is *too weak* to hold you to the diet, will in a few weeks begin to feel lighter and more youthful.

Remember this important fact—this diet will not starve you down. It is scientifically adequate and you will not lose weight at the cost of the constant feeling of hunger or sag lines in the face and throat, nor will your nerves be frayed and your disposition ruined. This is Food for

Beauty, not a routine of self-denial. Literally, you will eat your way to better body tone and loss of fat. Adhere to this diet until you lose enough pounds to bring you to the normal weight-height balance for your age. After that, go on to the 1,500 calorie diet for a month and after that go onto the maintenance diet permanently.

Your luncheon each day must consist of a large bowl of mixed greens plus grated raw vegetables or fresh fruit, served with a reducing dressing. (See recipe, page 110.) Before this vibrant salad bowl, take a 5 oz. glass of fresh fruit or vegetable juice, and after the bowl, a hot cup of clear saltless bouillon made from green vegetables.

One slice of melba or dry toast goes with your luncheon and one pat of margarine.

Yes, this special 800 calorie diet, which the short and heavy woman must follow until she resumes her more appealing feminine lines, is a fairly strict diet. Strict, but beneficial, remember. In presenting the 800 calorie diet, the four market seasons are taken into consideration, so you will not have any excuse to break the rules. Each menu is given as an example of the kind of menu you are to follow every day while you are on this diet.

FALL

—800 calories

BREAKFAST

1 bunch Concord grapes
1 slice melba toast
margarine
coffee without cream or sugar

LUNCHEON

The raw fruit or vegetable salad bowl
luncheon as described on page 95

DINNER

mixed fresh fruit salad
reducing dressing
garden bouillon
broiled calves liver
1 strip lean crisp bacon
Swiss chard   baked tomato
1 slice melba toast
margarine
black coffee

WINTER

—800 calories

BREAKFAST

½ grapefruit
1 slice melba toast
margarine
cream or sugar

EON

able salad bowl
ed on page 95

ER

l carrot salad
sing
leeks
f
nips

fresh fruit cup
black coffee

SPRING

—800 calories

BREAKFAST

*1 serving fresh strawberries
without sugar or cream
1 slice melba toast
margarine
coffee or tea without cream or sugar*

LUNCHEON

*The raw fruit or vegetable salad bowl
luncheon as described on page 95*

DINNER

*grapefruit and watercress salad
reducing dressing
essence of fresh tomatoes
½ broiled chicken
fresh asparagus
1 slice melba toast
margarine
raw apple
black coffee*

SUMMER

BREAKFAST

5 oz. orange juice
1 slice melba toast
margarine
coffee or tea without cream or sugar

LUNCHEON

The raw fruit or vegetable salad bowl
luncheon as described on page 95

DINNER

hearts of lettuce with green pepper rings
with or without reducing dressing
essence of fresh celery
1 broiled thick loin lamb chop
with lamb kidney
zucchini   carrots
both with melted margarine
1 slice melba toast
fresh raspberries
black coffee

The raw fruit or vegetable salad bowl luncheons suggested in above menus may be alternated with one of the *matière vivante* plates described in the chapter on recipes. It should be understood that the menus given here are to help you plan others like them, using the fruits and vegetables in your local markets at the time. The more you vary the ingredients, the more interesting and pleasant to follow will be any of these sunlight-nutrition diets. But no matter how you vary them, they must be kept within the caloric limits and at least half of the daily food allowance must consist of raw fresh fruits and vegetables.

On this 800 calorie diet, two glasses of skimmed milk or fresh buttermilk are allowed each day. One should be reserved for bedtime, the other for the between-meal hunger which might tempt you to nibble on forbidden sweets. An extra glass of grapefruit juice or orange juice can be added to the daily allowance if taken at 10:00 A.M. or 4:00 P.M. as a bracer.

Some women who are short find that they put on weight very quickly. But they take too much justifiable pride in their figures to allow the beauty-destroying excess weight to gain much headway. For them, the 800 calorie diet is a little too strict. A 1,000 calorie diet is all they need to keep their figures streamlined.

The tall woman who finds that she is getting heavy above the waist, should follow the 1,000 calorie diet also, especially if her weight is much above height-weight. However, for the tall woman with merely a few pounds too much, the 1,200 calorie diet is suggested. The low calorie content of a reducing diet is of course very important. But equally important is the faithfulness with which you follow it. Food for Beauty must be seasoned with the strong will to achieve its purpose, remember.

Luncheon on the 1,000 calorie diet menu is the same as on the 800 calorie diet menu, being either a large bowl of raw fruit or vegetable salad, preceded by a 5 oz. glass of fresh vegetable or fruit juice, and followed by a cup of hot clear vegetable bouillon, with fruit for dessert.

FALL

—1,000 calories

BREAKFAST

5 oz. grapefruit juice
1 soft-boiled egg
margarine
coffee or tea without cream or sugar

10 A.M.   *glass tomato juice*

LUNCHEON

Same as for 800 calorie menu

DINNER

lettuce, chicory, and watercress salad
reducing dressing
essence of celery root
1 small serving roast duck
applesauce sweetened with saccharine
Brussels sprouts
melon cup with lime juice and sprig
of fresh mint
black coffee

BEDTIME   *1 glass buttermilk*

WINTER

—1,000 calories

BREAKFAST

5 oz. orange juice
2 strips crisp lean bacon
1 slice melba toast
margarine
coffee or tea without cream or sugar

10 A.M. *glass carrot and pineapple juice*

LUNCHEON

Same as for 800 calorie menu

DINNER

salad of lettuce with grated raw
broccoli and yellow squash
reducing dressing
essence of fresh mushrooms
broiled lean steak
string beans
½ grapefruit
black coffee

BEDTIME *1 glass skim milk*

SPRING

—1,000 calories

BREAKFAST

1 serving fresh strawberries
small pitcher light cream
1 slice melba toast
margarine
coffee or tea without cream or sugar

10 A.M.   1 glass fresh spinach juice

LUNCHEON

Same as for 800 calorie menu

DINNER

lettuce and celery root salad
reducing dressing
herbal cream cheese balls
garden bouillon
½ broiled chicken
broccoli   new beets
fresh fruit cup
black coffee

BEDTIME   5 oz. orange juice

SUMMER

—1,000 calories

BREAKFAST

1 fresh peach sliced
small pitcher light cream
2 slices melba toast
margarine
coffee or tea without cream or sugar

10 A.M.   *1 glass vegetable juice*

LUNCHEON

Same as for 800 calorie menu

DINNER

lettuce, honeydew and cantaloupe salad
reducing dressing
herbal bouillon
baked squab
new peas   diced white squash
whole strawberries
black coffee

BEDTIME   *5 oz. skim milk*

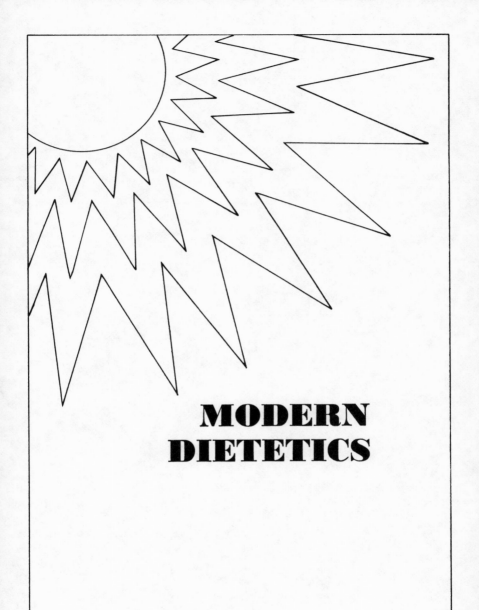

MODERN
DIETETICS

By now you have learned that Food for
Beauty is based on the sane and practical theories of
modern dietetics. In the Zurich Room of my salon in
New York dieticians with impeccable university and hos-
pital experience have for a long time been perfecting the
recipes which embody all the world-renowned theories of
Bircher-Benner. We have gone much further, for we
have adapted his ideas to the American temperament and
taste.

If you have been convinced that this vitalizing diet

of raw fruits and vegetables is what you need to rebuild your vitality and normalize your figure back to its intended youthfulness, then you must begin to learn how to prepare these raw fruits and vegetables in your own kitchen. Though they are served uncooked, they are served most attractively. In fact, so beautiful and appetite-appealing can sunlight foods be made, that the preparation of the dishes has developed into an art. It is an art which any woman can easily master.

In all the menus given for slenderizing, reducing dressing or mayonnaise has been recommended. The following recipes have been used in the Zurich Room where many of the wealthiest and most beautiful women of the world have followed the diets given in this book.

REDUCING DRESSING
(1 PINT)

1½ cups vegetable oil
½ cup strained lemon juice
1 teaspoon salt
2 saccharine tablets
½ egg yolk
1 small sliver of fresh garlic if desired

Combine ingredients and shake well. The garlic is important for both its flavor and its healthful qualities. The amount of garlic used can be increased to taste.

REDUCING MAYONNAISE

1 *egg yolk*
1 *cup vegetable oil*
1 *tablespoon lemon juice*
  salt to taste

Chill a small mixing bowl. Chill also the egg yolk, lemon juice, and oil. Use a chilled rotary egg beater. Place egg yolk, lemon juice, and salt into bowl. Beat well. Then add oil, a little at a time, beginning with about ½ teaspoon, and gradually increasing the amounts added. Beat well between additions of oil. Continue alternately to add oil and to beat well until a thick salad dressing is formed.

NOTE: If reducing mayonnaise separates, beat up another egg yolk or use a tablespoon of lemon juice or a tablespoon of water, and add the mayonnaise to it a little at a time, beating continuously.

For the normalizing sunlight diet, a reducing dressing is not necessary. The following recipe for French

111

dressing is given because so many clients have praised it
and begged for the recipe, which is given here for the
first time.

ZURICH ROOM
FRENCH DRESSING

1½ cups olive oil
½   cup lemon juice
1   teaspoon salt
2   teaspoons sugar
1   egg yolk
½   clove of garlic if desired

Combine salt and sugar with just enough lemon juice to
dissolve. Add egg yolk and beat with rotary beater until
mixture is fluffy. Then slowly beat in olive oil and remainder of lemon juice. Add garlic if desired. Let stand
in sealed jar in refrigerator.

In the reducing menus, various types of dry toast
have been suggested. Melba toast is easily made at home.
There are several delicious rusks, "reducing" cookies, and
wafers on the market. Zurich Toast is a flavorsome reducing specialty perfected by the dieticians of the Zurich
Room for the *matière vivante* luncheons. It is made of rye

flour, vegetable salts, and imported seeds indicated for reducing diets.

For the normalizing diets, health nut bread is suggested. The following is the prized secret recipe which has been begged for by countless visitors to the Zurich Room. It is also highly recommended for growing children.

ZURICH NUT BREAD

1 *cup rye flour*
⅔ *cup pastry flour*
2 *teaspoons baking powder*
⅓ *teaspoon salt*
½ *cup coarsely chopped walnuts*
½ *cup raw brown sugar*
1⅓ *cups buttermilk*
¾ *teaspoon baking soda*

Sift rye flour, pastry flour, baking powder, and salt together. Dust chopped nuts lightly with flour. Add a small amount of warm water to brown sugar, stir until smooth, then stir in buttermilk. Add baking soda to buttermilk mixture. Then quickly combine dry and liquid ingredients. Add nuts and mix well. Pour into well-greased bread

tins and bake in slow oven (300° F.) for 45 minutes.
Serve the following day.

Cream cheese and nuts are an excellent source of the
protein which is needed in any sound diet. By serving a
little herbal cheese mixture with the large fruit and vegetable plate or salad bowl, you will incorporate into the
meal the balancing requirement of protein.

HERBAL CREAM CHEESE MIXTURE

1 *pound fresh cream cheese*
1½ *teaspoons chopped fresh tarragon*
6 *oz. finely chopped nuts*

Combine and serve in a bowl or shape into small balls.
In all the menus, a herbal bouillon or vegetable essence
is recommended. You will note that this clear hot broth is
to be taken after the large service of raw fruits and vegetables in the luncheon menus, not before. You must never
lose sight of the fact that raw fruits and vegetables are the
major factors in this modern diet for health and beauty.
Everything else is secondary. Therefore, the hot soups,
important as they are with their mineral salts, are to be
taken only after the large amounts of nutritive fruits and
vegetables have been eaten.

114

The clear vegetable bouillons are very easy to make and achieve exceptionally rich flavor, despite their meat-lessness. They are really nothing more complicated than strained stock made of greens and vegetables carefully brewed. You will find for yourself ever changing combinations of lettuce leaves, celery stalks and tops, fresh vegetables, and herbs which will produce delightful mineral-rich bouillons. The recipes given below are merely to serve as examples.

HERBAL BOUILLON

1 *bunch green celery tops*
6 *outside lettuce leaves*
2 *large unpeeled carrots*
1 *large scrubbed unpeeled potato*
2 *leeks (entire)*
2 *tomatoes*
2 *quarts cold water*

Wash vegetables thoroughly. Cut up coarsely. Place in large enamel, copper, or glass kettle. Cover with cold water. Cover. Simmer for 2 hours. Then mash through fine sieve, season with salt and if desired, a few drops of lemon juice and serve hot in bouillon cups.

ESSENCE OF
FRESH MUSHROOM

2 *pounds unpeeled fresh mushrooms*
10 *outside lettuce leaves*
1 *large unpeeled carrot*
1 *leek (entire)*
1 *peeled potato*
2 *quarts cold water*

Wash vegetables thoroughly. Cut up fine. Place in large enamel, copper, or glass kettle. Cover with cold water. Cover. Simmer 2 hours. Then mash through fine sieve, season with salt and serve hot in bouillon cups.

ESSENCE OF GARDEN PEAS

1½ *pounds unshelled peas*
6 *outside lettuce leaves*
1 *bunch celery tops*
1 *leek (entire)*
1 *small peeled potato*
1 *small unpeeled carrot*
2 *sprigs parsley*
2 *quarts cold water*

116

Wash vegetables thoroughly. Do not shell peas. Cut up other vegetables coarsely. Place in large enamel, copper or glass kettle. Cover with cold water. Cover kettle. Simmer for 2 hours. Then mash through fine strainer. Season with salt. Serve hot in bouillon cups.

GARDEN BOUILLON

½ *pound string beans*
1 *summer squash*
1 *small cucumber*
3 *firm radishes*
1 *bunch watercress*
6 *outside lettuce leaves*
3 *outside celery stalks*
½ *bunch parsley*
2 *small white onions*
1 *turnip*
1 *carrot*
2 *quarts cold water*

Wash vegetables thoroughly but do not peel them. Cut up coarsely. Place in large enamel, copper, or glass kettle. Cover with cold water. Cover kettle. Simmer for 2 hours, then mash through fine sieve. Season with salt. Serve hot in bouillon cups.

ESSENCE OF TOMATO

2 *pounds ripe tomatoes*
1 *bunch green celery tops*
2 *leeks (entire)*
1 *small potato*
6 *outside lettuce leaves*
1 *cup empty pea pods*
2 *quarts cold water*

Wash vegetables thoroughly but do not peel them. Chop coarsely. Place in large enamel, copper, or glass kettle. Cover with cold water. Cover kettle. Simmer for 2 hours. Then mash through fine sieve. Serve hot in bouillon cups.

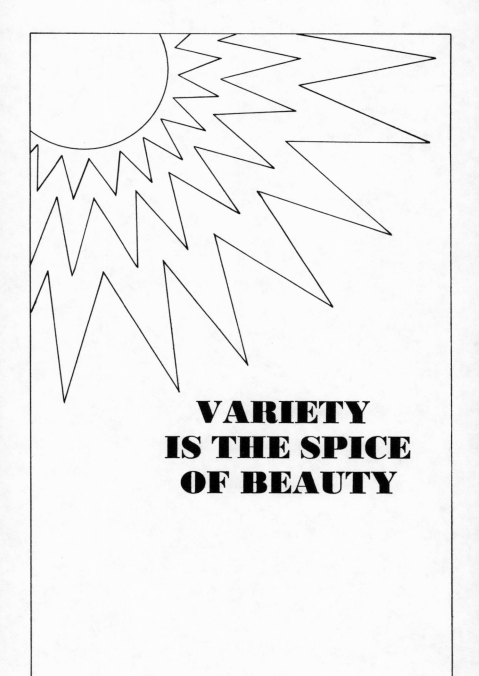

**VARIETY
IS THE SPICE
OF BEAUTY**

Imagine yourself entering an art gallery. At the door the curator stops you and asks that you listen for a second while he explains the purposes and significance behind the masterpieces you are about to see. "But we want only art, not a lecture," you exclaim.

In much the same way the reader enters this section of the book in which she expects to find nothing but recipes for the *matière vivante* luncheons which have become well known all over the world. I ask you to pause at the threshold while you listen to a short talk on the significance to you that lies behind those brilliant and sparkling arrangements of raw fruits and vegetables. They are not part of some diet fad. They are factors in a new way of living. When you have realized their importance in health and continued youthfulness to you and to your entire family, I am certain that the recipes will become matters of vital significance. Their fresh and gardenlike loveliness will delight the eye. Their surprising array of unsuspected flavors and consistencies will startle your palate. And after a little while, when you have learned to incorporate these foods into your diet, you will find that their dewy beauty in some mysterious way imparts to your body a quickened sense of living.

To the woman who dreads calories as much as she dreads the marks of years upon her face, raw fruits and vegetables are reassuring friends. They contain a negligible amount of calories in appetite-satisfying bulk. You can eat great servings of them without adding an extra pound to your own body. Yes, they will fill you up and give you the pleasant sensation of having eaten all you want without having run up the calorie overbalance. And because these raw fruits and vegetables have harmlessly satisfied your craving for food, they have spared you the temptation of nibbling at more concentrated foods in which calories are packed in terrifying amounts. Remember that fact as you read the recipes for Peach Solstice or Tropical Dawn, for example. Beautiful food! Yes, but also Food for Beauty.

Remember also as you read on through lists of garden and orchard ingredients that these blessings not only taste good and look colorful, but that they also contain much water. Water is something most of our daily diets lack. We forget that living tissues need large amounts of water to keep them healthy. In the large quantity of fruits and vegetables you henceforth will eat every day, there will literally be springs of fresh water to give your body the life-renewing baths which wash away the residues and toxins that threaten its youthful vitality. The large amount of water-bearing fruits and vegetables you will learn to eat will insure you against dehydration of body tissues and supply your kidneys with liquids that the kidneys demand if they are to throw off the waste that is their function to dispose of.

Those beautiful raw foods which must constitute at least half of your daily ration have other essential virtues. They carry in their tender tissues the metallic ions needed to keep your blood normal, thereby sustaining a normal acid-base balance in the body. Vitamins in prodigal amounts are supplied by these raw fruits and vegetables. "But do not cooked vegetables contain all the vitamins we need?" Let me quote Dr. Walter H. Eddy of Columbia University in answer. "When you are told that 2 oz. of raw cabbage contain about as much Vitamin C as 40 oz. of boiled cabbage, you will appreciate the value of the raw product." He adds a statement which will surprise many orange and tomato enthusiasts. "What few seem to know is that vegetables such as cabbage and salad greens are almost equally rich sources (of Vitamin C) and can well be used to satisfy the desire for variety."

Variety is of tremendous importance in the Food for Beauty Diet. One or two raw vegetables are not enough. Nor is one kind of fruit or fruit juice enough. The *matière vivante* luncheons as served in the Zurich Room consist each of a minimum of 21 *different* raw fruits and vegetables. Of course it is not practical for the woman to try for such great variety in her own home unless she has a staff of assistants. She must, however, use at least 6 different fruits and vegetables each meal.

There are two reasons for this need of wide variety. You, as an individual, have an individual skin. If your skin is to remain soft and clear and beautiful, the derma, or basic skin, must be perfectly normal—that is, it must maintain perfect health. The health of your skin depends on many factors, vitamins and minerals being among the most important. But what minerals and what vitamins and in what amounts does your own individual skin need to keep it normal? No conscientious dermatologist would claim to know the answer. But he would advise you to eat as wide a variety of minerals and vitamins as possible, so that your food can contain such a wide margin of all the vitamins and minerals that your skin's individual requirements for derma-health can be supplied. That will explain why Bircher-Benner and I lay such stress on many different fruits and vegetables in the daily diet for

124

the woman who realizes that balanced health is the framework of which radiant beauty is built.

This can be stated in another way. The B-complex vitamin maintains normal activity of the digestive system. A variety of foods guarantees the supply of ingredients from which B-complex vitamin can be made. I quote the great American nutrition authority Dr. Walter H. Eddy to explain in further detail the B-complex vitamin in relation to raw fruits and vegetables. Dr. Eddy writes in *Good Housekeeping Magazine* for September 1938: "As study of the B-complex has gone on, we have discovered that nature put into the B-complex quite a variety of separate vitamin factors, and that these factors have a definite interdependence. It must be remembered, however, that man's identification of the factors nature puts into foodstuffs has been slow and is still probably far from complete. Natural sources of vitamins may thus give us combinations that man has yet been unable to duplicate exactly.

"So I would again urge the more general use of raw vegetables. By eating them in the raw state we preserve all their inherent complex qualities; we take no chance of destroying any of those qualities through cooking. In the raw state, vegetables also provide abundance of resistance-building Vitamin A."

The recipes given here are for 4 servings each. They are the ones used in the Zurich Room in New York and have proved highly successful with both men and women.

125

It is true, they are Food for Beauty in the full meaning of that phrase. But they are important also in the regular menus of any home where the maintenance of health and the need of building modern food habits are intelligently recognized. Therefore I urge the woman who realizes the need to slenderize to use these recipes not only for that important purpose. I urge her to serve these *matière vivante* dishes to her husband and her children as well. In Switzerland I have seen *entire families* thrive on this food. Yes, even very young children. And nowhere else will you find *sturdier* young girls and boys.

Now we can enter the gallery knowing in advance the significance of all we shall see. Before us stretch acres of gardens. Peas, beans, carrots, turnips, and squashes of many kinds thrive in the sunlight. Apples redden in the orchard, pears grow ruddy, grapes ripen on leafy vines, and purple plums grow fat.

Sunlight food! Infinite variety. Flavors and consistencies that are countless. This is the stuff of youth and beauty, this is Food for Beauty that is based on abundant health.

In another chapter the way to use these *matière vivante* plates in your family menus is discussed. For women on stricter diets than the 2,500 calorie maintenance diet, use one of these plates as the main meal of the day, at the usual time you are in the habit of eating your main meal.

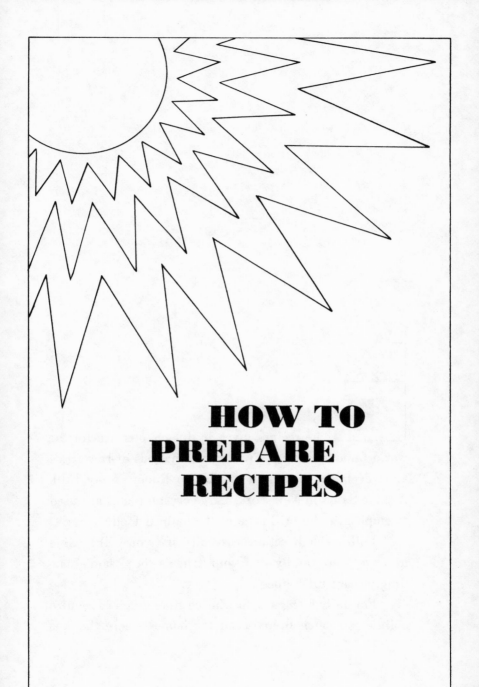

HOW TO
PREPARE
RECIPES

The recipes given in this chapter are for the world famous *matière vivante* combinations of raw fruits and vegetables served in the Zurich Room of my Fifth Avenue Salon in New York. Large crystal plates are used to emphasize the brilliance of the natural food.

Follow the directions carefully and you will be able to serve your family and your friends these same startlingly beautiful recipes.

For daily home use, the Zurich Room recipes require a little too much preparation for homes where there is not a large staff. The second recipe for each dish is given for women who have neither servant nor much time for preparing food. The domestic version will not be as elaborate as the Zurich Room dish, but it will be adequate from every nutritional viewpoint and will also be delicious and interesting.

Clean the vegetables with great care. Scrub and wash them but do not peel. They are to be grated, chopped, or sliced and cut according to each recipe's requirement. Chill the fruits, vegetables, and greens well. It makes them more crisp and pleasant to eat.

SUNSWEPT CRESCENT

(4 INDIVIDUAL MATIÈRE VIVANTE PLATES)

AS PREPARED IN THE ZURICH ROOM

INGREDIENTS

1 *medium size honeydew*
1 *large grapefruit*
1 *large orange*
½ *cup of strawberries*
8 *red cherries with stems*
½ *cup of herbal cream cheese mixture*
1 *lime*
2 *tablespoons of shelled peas*
¼ *bunch of watercress*
¼ *pound of lima beans*
½ *yellow turnip*
1 *carrot*
½ *white squash*
1 *cucumber*
4 *large radishes*
1 *small yellow squash*
4 *small pieces of celery*
4 *pieces of chicory*
12 *small lettuce cups*

METHOD

Cut honeydew into quarters lengthwise. Using sharp knife, run it from one end to the other as near rind as possible to free fruit without taking it off the ring. Then cut downward to the rind in evenly spaced slices to make the melon easier to eat.

Remove perfect sections from grapefruit and orange. Clean strawberries and slice lengthwise. Pit cherries and stuff with herbal cream cheese mixture. Slice lime into quarters.

Chop peas, watercress, lima beans. Grate turnip, carrot, white squash, cucumber, radish, yellow squash. Cut chicory with sharp scissors.

In center of large plate, place the honeydew quarter. Sprinkle a little cut chicory over melon, then lay sections of grapefruit and orange alternately along the melon, placing them diagonally. Between slices of grapefruit and orange place slices of strawberry, and over top sprinkle finely chopped green peas. Near the honeydew, place a slice of lime.

Place 3 lettuce cups around edge of plate at equal distances. Between them place the 2 stuffed cherries and the single piece of crisp celery stuffed with chopped watercress.

Fill the three lettuce cups lightly as follows:

1. grated turnip, grated carrot and grated white squash.
2. grated yellow squash and chopped lima beans.
3. grated cucumber and grated radish.

131

SUNSWEPT CRESCENT

(4 SERVINGS)

THE SAME RECIPE SIMPLIFIED FOR YOUR HOME

INGREDIENTS

  1 *large honeydew*
  1 *large orange*
  1 *large grapefruit*
12 *large cherries*
½ *cup herbal cream cheese mixture*
  1 *lime*
  2 *large cucumbers*
  4 *small carrots*
  2 *large lettuce leaves*
12 *small lettuce cups*
  1 *tablespoon ground walnuts*

METHOD

Cut honeydew into quarters lengthwise. Using sharp knife, run it from one end to the other as near the rind as possible to free fruit without taking it off the ring. Then cut downward to the rind in evenly spaced slices to make the melon easier to eat.

Remove perfect sections from orange and grapefruit. Pit cherries and stuff with herbal cream cheese mixture. Slice lime into quarters. Grate cucumbers and carrots. Shred lettuce leaves.

In center of a large plate place the honeydew quarter. Over the melon sprinkle a little shredded lettuce. Then lay sections of orange and grapefruit alternately along melon, placing them diagonally. Near the melon place a slice of lime.

Place 3 lettuce cups around edge of plate at equal distances. Between them put 3 stuffed cherries.

Fill the three lettuce cups lightly as follows:

1. grated carrot garnished with walnuts.
2. grated cucumber.
3. mixture of grated carrot and cucumber.

JADE IN SUNLIGHT

(4 INDIVIDUAL MATIÈRE VIVANTE PLATES)

AS PREPARED IN THE ZURICH ROOM

INGREDIENTS

1 *large avocado*
1 *grapefruit*
½ *cup strawberries*
¼ *cup blanched almonds*
1 *red plum*
8 *red grapes*
¼ *cup herbal cream cheese mixture*
½ *large orange*
¼ *pound peas*
½ *green pepper*
¼ *cup spinach*
¼ *pound lima beans*
1 *small crooked neck squash*
¼ *zucchini*
8 *radishes*
½ *turnip*
12 *lettuce cups*
1 *tablespoon chopped pistachio nuts*

METHOD

Peel avocado and slice lengthwise into quarters. Sprinkle with lemon or other fruit juice to prevent discoloration. Peel grapefruit and remove sections.

Clean strawberries and cut crosswise into thick slices. Cut almonds in half. Slice unpeeled plum into quarters. Remove seeds from grapes and stuff with herbal cream cheese mixture. Peel orange and cut crosswise into thick slices. Cut each thick slice in half. Next, cut a slit into each half section of orange and into the slit stuff some chopped green peas.

Chop pepper, spinach, lima beans, peas. Grate squash, zucchini, radishes, turnip. Cut celery into thin slices.

In center of large dish, place avocado quarter. Lay 2 perfect sections of grapefruit lengthwise in avocado. Between grapefruit slices place thick slices of strawberry and almond halves.

Arrange 3 lettuce cups around edge of plate. Between them place the 2 stuffed grapes and the pea-filled fan-shaped orange.

Fill the 3 lettuce cups lightly as follows:

1. grated squash, celery slices, chopped pepper, chopped pistachio nuts.
2. grated zucchini, small amount of grated radish, and one plum quarter.
3. grated turnip, chopped lima beans, and chopped spinach.

135

JADE IN SUNLIGHT

(4 SERVINGS)

THE SAME RECIPE SIMPLIFIED FOR YOUR HOME

INGREDIENTS

2 *medium size avocadoes*
2 *large lettuce leaves*
1 *grapefruit*
½ *cup strawberries*
2 *white turnips (large)*
1 *zucchini*
1 *pear*
12 *lettuce cups*
4 *herbal cream cheese balls*

METHOD

Peel avocadoes and sprinkle with any fruit juice to prevent discoloration.

Cut large lettuce leaves very fine. Peel grapefruit and section. Hull strawberries, slice lengthwise. Peel white turnip and grate. Wash zucchini and grate.

Place pear in center of plate, fill with shredded lettuce and then lay in grapefruit sections so they form a flowerlike appearance. Between sections place sliced strawberries so they give a decorative appearance.

Place 3 lettuce cups on plate. Fill them lightly as follows with:

1. grated turnip.
2. an herbal cream cheese ball covered with zucchini.
3. a mixture of turnip and zucchini.

PERSIMMON SOLSTICE

(4 INDIVIDUAL MATIÈRE VIVANTE PLATES)

AS PREPARED IN THE ZURICH ROOM

INGREDIENTS

4 *persimmons*
1 *small pineapple*
12 *large grapes*
¼ *cup herbal cream cheese mixture*
1 *slice honeydew*
4 *cherry tomatoes*
½ *head cauliflower*
1 *green pepper (small)*
¼ *pound lima beans*
¼ *bunch parsley*
½ *cabbage*
1 *small crooked neck squash*
1 *zucchini*
1 *carrot*
4 *large lettuce cups*
12 *romaine cups*

METHOD

Peel persimmons and cut in half. Sprinkle with fruit juice. Dice pineapple. Pit grapes and stuff with herbal cream cheese mixture. Scoop small balls from honeydew. Slice cherry tomatoes. Chop cauliflower, green pepper, lima beans, parsley, cabbage. Grate squash, zucchini, carrot.

In center of plate, place large lettuce cup made of two crisp leaves. In lettuce cup, arrange chopped cabbage, then diced pineapple piled high. On the pineapple mound, lay one persimmon half, concave side down, and one half concave side up. Garnish liberally with chopped green pepper.

Around edge of plate, arrange 3 neatly trimmed romaine cups. Between the cups place stuffed Belgian grapes. Fill the romaine cups lightly as follows:

1. grated zucchini and slices of cherry tomato.
2. grated squash and chopped lima beans garnished with chopped parsley.
3. chopped cauliflower, grated carrot, a second light layer of chopped cauliflower garnished with small melon balls.

PERSIMMON SOLSTICE

(4 SERVINGS)

THE SAME RECIPE SIMPLIFIED FOR YOUR HOME

INGREDIENTS

  4 *persimmons*
  ½ *head cabbage*
  1 *small pineapple*
  2 *white squash (medium sized)*
  4 *large herbal cream cheese balls*
  1 *very large yellow turnip*
  4 *large lettuce cups*
  1 *green pepper*
12 *medium size lettuce cups*
  1 *tablespoon ground pistachio nuts*

METHOD

Peel persimmon, cut in half and sprinkle with fruit juice.

Chop cabbage very fine. Peel pineapple and dice. Scrub squash and grate. Peel turnip and grate.

In center of the plate make a large lettuce cup, fill with cabbage and diced pineapple. On top place the 2 persimmon halves, one concave side down and one concave side up. If you have any green pepper, chop it and use for a garnish.

Place 3 lettuce cups on plate, fill lightly as follows:

1. grated white squash.
2. grated turnip with a garnish of pistachio.
3. squash and turnip which have been well blended. In this cup, first put the herbal cream cheese ball and cover with mixture.

SUNSWEPT ONYX

(4 INDIVIDUAL MATIÈRE VIVANTE PLATES)

AS PREPARED IN THE ZURICH ROOM

INGREDIENTS

½ cantaloupe
¼ pound red cherries
20 large blackberries
¼ mango
¼ head cabbage
¼ bunch parsley
¼ bunch watercress
   a few celery leaves
½ bunch broccoli
¼ pound peas
½ head cauliflower
1 carrot
1 small crooked neck squash
8 radishes
1 beet
1 cup herbal cream cheese mixture
16 lettuce cups

METHOD

Peel cantaloupe and slice into 16 half-moon strips. Slice cherries. Clean blackberries. Cut mango into quarters.

Chop cabbage, parsley, watercress, celery leaves, broccoli, peas, cauliflower. Grate carrot, squash, radishes, beets. Make five small herbal cream cheese balls.

In center of large plate, make circle of 5 large blackberries and 5 herbal cream cheese balls.

Fill center with sliced cherries. Around edge of plate, arrange 4 lettuce cups and between them place half moons of cantaloupe, all lying parallel to each other.

Fill lettuce cups lightly as follows:

1. grated summer squash, chopped watercress, and section of mango.
2. grated carrot, chopped cabbage, and chopped parsley.
3. grated beets, chopped cauliflower, and chopped peas.
4. chopped broccoli and grated radishes.

SUNSWEPT ONYX

(4 SERVINGS)

THE SAME RECIPE SIMPLIFIED FOR YOUR HOME

INGREDIENTS

2 *large lettuce leaves*
¼ *pound red cherries*
1 *head cauliflower*
3 *large beets*
1 *cup herbal cream cheese mixture*
20 *large blackberries*
16 *lettuce cups*
2 *tablespoons walnuts (chopped fine)*

METHOD

Cut the 2 large leaves of lettuce in very fine pieces (like shreds). Slice cherries. Grate cauliflower. Peel and grate beets. Make 20 balls of the cheese the size of the blackberries.

In center of plate make a ring of 5 blackberries and between each two put a herbal cream cheese ball. Fill the center with shredded lettuce and sliced cherries.

Put 4 cups at regular intervals on plate. Fill 2 opposite with cauliflower and in the other 2 put beets. Garnish cauliflower with chopped nuts.

TROPICAL RADIANCE

(4 INDIVIDUAL MATIÈRE VIVANTE PLATES)

AS PREPARED IN THE ZURICH ROOM

INGREDIENTS

1 *bunch watercress*
¼ *pound peas*
¼ *head broccoli*
½ *head cauliflower*
1 *carrot*
1 *beet*
8 *radishes*
1 *small crooked neck squash*
½ *zucchini*
¼ *cup sliced strawberries*
1 *small ear corn*
4 *fresh figs*
24 *very small lettuce cups*
¼ *cup blackberries*

METHOD

Chop watercress, peas, broccoli, cauliflower. Grate carrot, beet, radishes, squash, zucchini. Slice strawberries and cut kernels from corn.

Slice figs into 8 sections each, but do not cut through. Push sections open to form a flower. Place flowered fig in center of large plate. Around edge of plate, arrange 6 lettuce cups at equal distances.

Fill each cup lightly as follows:

1. grated squash and chopped peas.
2. chopped watercress and sliced strawberries.
3. chopped broccoli and grated radish.
4. grated radish and kernels of corn.
5. chopped cauliflower and blackberries.
6. grated zucchini and grated beets.

TROPICAL RADIANCE

(4 SERVINGS)

THE SAME RECIPE SIMPLIFIED FOR YOUR HOME

INGREDIENTS

 4 *fresh figs*
 1 *large head of broccoli*
 2 *large white turnips*
 ½ *cup strawberries*
 16 *medium size lettuce cups*

METHOD

Cut fig so it looks like a flower and place it in center of the plate.

Grate the stem part of the broccoli and chop the flower part. Mix well together.

Wash turnip, peel and grate. Hull strawberries, slice crosswise.

Place 4 lettuce cups on plate at regular intervals. Fill 2 with grated turnip and on 1 of the turnip cups place sliced strawberries. Fill other 2 cups with broccoli.

APRICOT-GREEN
ALMOND SOLSTICE

(4 INDIVIDUAL MATIÈRE VIVANTE PLATES)

AS PREPARED IN THE ZURICH ROOM

INGREDIENTS

4 *large apricots*

½ *pound green almonds*

½ *head cabbage*

½ *head broccoli*

1 *green pepper*

1 *crooked neck squash*

1 *beet*

1 *small ear corn*

1 *small pineapple*

12 *cherries*

½ *cup herbal cream cheese mixture*

½ *cantaloupe*

¼ *cup strawberries*

4 *large lettuce cups*

12 *romaine cups*

4 *pieces of chicory*

150

METHOD

Scrub apricots and cut in half. Sprinkle with fruit juice. Shell almonds and blanch. Chop cabbage, broccoli, green pepper. Grate squash and beet. Scrape corn kernels from cob and chop fine. Dice pineapple. Pit cherries and stuff with herbal cream cheese. Scoop 8 balls from cantaloupe. Clean and slice strawberries.

In center of large plate, arrange a crisp large lettuce cup. Place a chicory sprig cut with scissors on bottom of cup, then a loose layer of chopped cabbage. Next a layer of diced pineapple. On top, place 2 apricot halves, one with concave side down, the other with concave side up. Fill the latter with chopped pepper and sliced green almonds.

Around edge of plate, arrange 3 romaine cups evenly spaced. Between the romaine cups place stuffed cherries.

Fill each romaine cup lightly as follows:

1. chopped broccoli and sliced strawberries.
2. grated squash and 2 cantaloupe balls.
3. grated beets and chopped corn.

APRICOT-GREEN ALMOND SOLSTICE

(4 SERVINGS)

THE SAME RECIPE SIMPLIFIED FOR YOUR HOME

INGREDIENTS

 4 *large apricots*
½ *head cabbage*
½ *pineapple*
½ *pound green almonds*
 1 *large zucchini*
 3 *large carrots*
 4 *large lettuce cups*
 4 *large herbal cream cheese balls*
12 *small lettuce cups*

METHOD

Scrub apricots, cut in half, remove pit, and sprinkle with fruit juice.

Chop cabbage very fine. Peel pineapple and dice. Shell almonds and blanch. Scrub zucchini and carrots and grate.

In center of plate put a large lettuce cup. Fill with first chopped cabbage and then pineapple. Make a mound and on top place the 2 apricot halves, one face down and the other up. On the one face up, put a herbal cream cheese ball and stick almonds into it.

Place 3 lettuce cups at regular intervals on plate. Fill each cup lightly as follows:

1. grated carrot.
2. grated zucchini.
3. carrot and zucchini which have been well blended.

TROPICAL DAWN

(4 INDIVIDUAL MATIÈRE VIVANTE PLATES)

AS PREPARED IN THE ZURICH ROOM

INGREDIENTS

1 *large pineapple*
½ *pound fresh dates*
1 *small box strawberries*
¼ *cup herbal cream cheese mixture*
¼ *bunch broccoli*
½ *zucchini*
¼ *turnip*
½ *summer squash*
1 *carrot*
4 *orange sections*
1 *tablespoon ground pistachio nuts*
½ *cauliflower*
8 *endive spears*
4 *Carlsbad plums*
4 *small lettuce leaves*
8 *small lettuce cups*
1 *tablespoon chopped almonds*

METHOD

Do not peel pineapple. Slice into quarters lengthwise, leaving a few of the spines on each quarter. Scoop out the pineapple, leaving only a pineapple shell.

Pit dates and cut into thin pieces. Clean strawberries and slice lengthwise. Stuff endive with herbal cream cheese mixture.

Grate stem of broccoli, zucchini, turnip, summer squash, carrot. Chop flower of broccoli, peas, cauliflower. Combine prepared broccoli and zucchini, turnip and carrot, summer squash and cauliflower, pineapple and dates.

Fill pineapple shell lightly with pineapple and date combination. Cover top with sliced strawberries. Arrange pineapple case in center of large plate with spears just over edge. On each side of pineapple, place a stuffed spear of endive. At base of pineapple, lay one Carlsbad plum on a small lettuce cup. On each side of the plum, but not too close, place a lettuce cup. Fill lightly as follows:

1. broccoli-zucchini mixture, turnip-carrot mixture, slice of orange sprinkled with pistachio nuts.
2. cauliflower-summer squash mixture, chopped peas and sprinkling of chopped almond.

TROPICAL DAWN

(4 SERVINGS)

THE SAME RECIPE SIMPLIFIED FOR YOUR HOME

INGREDIENTS

1 *large pineapple*
1 *pint box strawberries*
1 *large turnip*
1 *large zucchini*
1 *tablespoon ground pistachio nuts*
8 *herbal cream cheese balls*
8 *medium size lettuce cups*

METHOD

Cut pineapple into quarters lengthwise. Do not peel. Scoop out inside. Chop inside very fine and refill pine-apple. Hull strawberries and slice. Lay on top of pine-apple so the whole top is covered.

Grate turnip after it has been peeled. Wash zucchini and grate.

Lay pineapple in center of plate. Place 2 lettuce cups on either side. Fill one with turnip garnished with chopped pistachio nuts and the other with zucchini.

Place 2 herbal cream cheese balls between cups and pineapple.

LOTUS IN SUNLIGHT

(4 INDIVIDUAL MATIÈRE VIVANTE PLATES)

AS PREPARED IN THE ZURICH ROOM

INGREDIENTS

 4 *fresh figs*
 4 *pieces of chicory*
 1 *cup raspberries*
 ¼ *honeydew melon*
 ½ *pound of peas*
 ½ *bunch watercress*
 8 *leaves spinach*
 1 *carrot*
 1 *cucumber*
 8 *radishes*
 1 *beet*
 1 *small crooked neck squash*
 ½ *turnip*
20 *very small lettuce cups*
 8 *balls herbal cream cheese mixture*

METHOD

Slice figs into quarters, but do not cut all the way through. Fill figs with cut chicory and raspberries. From the honeydew melon, slice 20 flat strips about 3 inches long and ¾ inch wide.

Chop peas, watercress, spinach. Grate carrot, cucumber, radishes, beet, squash, turnip.

Place filled fig in center of large plate. Lay 5 melon strips on plate radiating from fig, at equal distances.

Between each 2 melon strips, place a lettuce cup.

Fill the lettuce cups lightly as follows:

1. grated yellow squash and chopped peas.
2. grated carrot and grated cucumber.
3. herbal cheese ball buried in grated radish.
4. chopped spinach, grated turnip and chopped watercress mixed together.
5. herbal cream cheese ball buried in grated beet.

LOTUS IN SUNLIGHT

(4 SERVINGS)

THE SAME RECIPE SIMPLIFIED FOR YOUR HOME

INGREDIENTS

4 *fresh figs*
¼ *honeydew melon*
½ *pound peas*
8 *spinach leaves*
1 *carrot*
1 *cucumber*
8 *radishes*
   a few raspberries (optional)
8 *small lettuce cups*
8 *herbal cream cheese balls*

METHOD

Slice figs into quarters, but do not cut all the way through.

From honeydew melon, slice 20 flat strips about 3 inches long and ¾ inch wide. Chop peas and spinach. Grate carrot and cucumber. Cut radishes into flowers.

Place cut fig in center of large plate. Place a few raspberries in center. Lay 5 melon strips on plate radiating from fig, at equal distances. Fill the 2 lettuce cups lightly as follows:

1. chopped spinach and chopped peas.
2. grated carrot and grated cucumber.

Between each 2 melon strips lay one of the following in order given: Filled lettuce cup, radish flower, lettuce cup, herbal cream cheese ball, radish flower.

L'AUBE FRAMBOISÉE

(RASPBERRY DAWN)

(4 INDIVIDUAL MATIÈRE VIVANTE PLATES)

AS PREPARED IN THE ZURICH ROOM

INGREDIENTS

  2 *small pineapples*
  1 *pound peas*
½ *small cabbage*
  1 *large green pepper*
½ *bunch watercress*
  1 *bunch radishes*
½ *white squash*
  1 *crooked neck squash*
  1 *zucchini*
  1 *beet*
  1 *pint raspberries*
12 *fresh dates*
½ *orange, rind and juice*
  8 *small stalks celery*
  4 *herbal cream cheese balls*
12 *small lettuce cups*
½ *pound lima beans*

METHOD

Slice pineapples in half, lengthwise, leaving on stem. Trim spines with scissors to give neat appearance. Scoop out centers. Chop scooped-out pineapple. Chop peas, cabbage, green pepper, and watercress, all very fine. Grate radishes, white squash, crooked neck squash, zucchini, and beet. Carefully wash and pick over the raspberries. Grind dates and mix with juice and rind of orange and make into 4 balls.

Stuff 4 stalks of celery with chopped watercress. Stuff the other 4 stalks of celery with grated radishes. In bottom of pineapple shell place a small amount of chopped cabbage. Beginning at the spine end of the pineapple, place a row of chopped peas, next a row of chopped pineapple, next a row of chopped cabbage, and finally a row of chopped green pepper.

Arrange the colorfully filled pineapple in the center of a large plate so that the spines just reach over the edge. On one side of the pineapple place a stalk of celery stuffed with watercress, next to it an herbal cream cheese ball. On the other side of the pineapple place a stalk of celery stuffed with radish and next to it a date ball. At the base of the pineapple arrange 3 lettuce cups close together.

Fill lightly as follows:

1. place grated yellow squash with a garnish of chopped lima beans.
2. grated white squash with a garnish of grated beets.
3. grated zucchini with a garnish of radish.

163

L'AUBE FRAMBOISÉE

(RASPBERRY DAWN)

(4 SERVINGS)

THE SAME RECIPE SIMPLIFIED FOR YOUR HOME

INGREDIENTS

2 *small pineapples*

½ *small cabbage*

1 *green pepper*

1 *large yellow squash*

3 *beets*

1 *pint of raspberries*

12 *small lettuce cups*

8 *herbal cream cheese balls*

METHOD

Slice pineapple in half lengthwise, leaving on stem. Trim spine with scissors to give neat appearance. Scoop out centers. Chop scooped-out pineapple. Chop cabbage and green pepper very fine. Grate squash and beets.

In bottom of pineapple place a little chopped cabbage. Beginning at spine end of pineapple place a row of chopped pepper, then a row of chopped pineapple, then a row of raspberries, then a row of chopped cabbage and lastly a row of chopped pepper.

Arrange this pineapple in the center of a large plate so that the spine just reaches over the edge of the plate. At the base of the pineapple place 3 lettuce cups together.

Fill cups lightly as follows:

1. place beets
2. place grated squash
3. place grated beets

On either side of pineapple place a herbal cream cheese ball.

CITRUS SUNWHEEL

(4 INDIVIDUAL MATIÈRE VIVANTE PLATES)

AS PREPARED IN THE ZURICH ROOM

INGREDIENTS

2 *large grapefruits*
8 *kumquats (fresh)*
8 *green grapes*
1 *tangerine*
3 *fresh figs*
1 *small head of cauliflower*
¼ *pound lima beans*
½ *cup chopped cabbage*
  a few celery leaves
¼ *bunch parsley*
½ *cup spinach*
2 *acorn squashes*
1 *cucumber*
1 *small yellow squash*
½ *bunch of mint*
12 *small lettuce cups*
¼ *cup herbal cream cheese mixture*

METHOD

Cut grapefruit in half. Remove center, then with sharp knife remove white membrane between the sections of fruit. Slice kumquats and seeded grapes. Peel tangerine and separate into sections, free of white parts. Cut each fig into quarters.

Chop cauliflower, lima beans, cabbage, celery leaves, parsley, spinach.

Grate acorn squash, cucumber, summer squash.

Between each two sections of prepared grapefruit, insert a slice of kumquat. In center of grapefruit, place a section of tangerine with 4 slices of grape. Garnish with fresh sprig of mint. Arrange the grapefruit in center of large plate.

Arrange 3 lettuce cups around edge of plate at equal distances. Between each 2 cups place a fig quarter. Using pastry tube, border one side of fig with moist herbal cream cheese mixture.

Fill the lettuce cups lightly as follows:

1. grated acorn squash, chopped spinach, and grated cucumber.
2. chopped cauliflower garnished with a few chopped lima beans and chopped celery leaves.
3. grated yellow squash and chopped cabbage mixed with chopped parsley.

CITRUS SUNWHEEL

(4 SERVINGS)

THE SAME RECIPE SIMPLIFIED FOR YOUR HOME

INGREDIENTS

2 *large grapefruits*
12 *kumquats*
1 *head of cauliflower*
3 *large carrots*
¼ *cup herbal cream cheese mixture*
12 *small lettuce cups*

METHOD

Cut grapefruit in half, remove center, then with a sharp knife remove white membrane between the sections. Slice 10 kumquats in thin slices. Cut 2 in half. Chop cauliflower. Grate carrot. Make 4 balls of herbal cream cheese mixture.

Between each two sections of prepared grapefruit insert 2 slices of kumquat. In center of grapefruit put a kumquat half. Place grapefruit in center of a salad plate.

Fill cups lightly as follows:

1. a herbal cheese ball sprinkled with carrots and garnished with cauliflower.
2. cauliflower garnished with carrot.
3. mixture of cauliflower and carrot, well blended.

PLUM SOLSTICE

(4 INDIVIDUAL MATIÈRE VIVANTE PLATES)

AS PREPARED IN THE ZURICH ROOM

INGREDIENTS

  4 *large red plums*
  1 *cup herbal cream cheese mixture*
  1 *grapefruit*
  1 *apricot*
12 *fresh dates*
  1 *small pineapple*
  4 *pieces of chicory*
½ *head of cabbage*
½ *green pepper*
¼ *pound peas*
¼ *pound lima beans*
¼ *bunch parsley*
½ *turnip*
½ *crooked neck squash*
  1 *carrot*
  1 *large cucumber*
  8 *radishes*
  4 *large lettuce cups*
¼ *cup blanched almonds*
12 *small romaine cups*

170

METHOD

Cut plums in half. Remove pits. Sprinkle with fruit juice. Using part of herbal cream cheese mixture, make 4 small balls. Peel and cut grapefruit into perfect sections. Cut apricot into 4 sections. Pit dates and stuff with herbal cream cheese. Dice pineapple, cut chicory fine.

Chop cabbage, green pepper, peas, lima beans, parsley. Grate turnips, squash, carrot, cucumber, radish.

In center of large plate, place large lettuce cup. In bottom, lightly place ¼ cup chopped cabbage, then heap with diced pineapple. On top of pineapple, place 2 plum halves, one with concave side down, one with concave side up and fill with herbal cream cheese ball. Stick cheese ball with almond slices. Garnish this center cup with chopped pepper.

Place the 3 romaine cups around edge of plate at equal distances. Between each 2 romaine cups, place a stuffed date.

Fill romaine cups lightly as follows:

1. grated turnip, chopped peas, a few chopped lima beans, and garnish with apricot section.
2. grated summer squash, grated carrot, and chopped parsley.
3. grated cucumber, grated radish, and grapefruit sections.

PLUM SOLSTICE

(4 SERVINGS)

THE SAME RECIPE SIMPLIFIED FOR YOUR HOME

INGREDIENTS

4 *large red plums*
1 *small pineapple*
½ *green pepper*
1 *small head of cabbage*
1 *head of broccoli*
2 *large beets*
4 *large lettuce cups*
4 *herbal cream cheese balls*
¼ *cup blanched almonds*
16 *small lettuce cups*

METHOD

Cut plums in half. Remove pits. Sprinkle with fruit juice. Peel pineapple and dice. Chop green pepper and chop cabbage both very fine. Chop the flower of the broccoli, grate the stem, and mix the two together. Peel beet and grate.

In center of a plate place large lettuce cup. Fill with cabbage and pineapple. On top place 2 plum halves, one concave side down and one concave side up. In the one which is concave side up, place the herbal cream cheese ball and stick with blanched almonds which have been split in half. Garnish with chopped pepper.

Fill cups lightly as follows:

1. beets garnished with broccoli.
2. broccoli garnished with a very little beet.
3. broccoli and beet well blended.

SUN STAR

(4 INDIVIDUAL MATIÈRE VIVANTE PLATES)

AS PREPARED IN THE ZURICH ROOM

INGREDIENTS

- 2 grapefruits
- 1 persimmon
- 1 green pepper
- 4 black grapes
- 2 tangerines
- 1 cup herbal cream cheese mixture
- ¼ cup pistachio nuts
- ½ head broccoli
- ¼ head cabbage
- ¼ bunch parsley
- ¼ pound peas
- 1 crooked neck squash
- 1 cucumber
- 1 carrot
- ½ turnip
- 4 kumquats
- 16 small lettuce cups

METHOD

Peel grapefruit and remove 8 perfect sections. Slice thin sections from persimmon. Cut thin strips of green pepper. Cut gash into fat edge of each grapefruit section. Then insert persimmon section into the gash. On each side of persimmon, insert strip of green pepper.

Slice black grapes. Peel tangerine. Separate into sections. Make 8 small herbal cream cheese balls and 4 large herbal cream cheese balls. Chop pistachio nuts and roll large cheese balls in chopped nuts.

Chop broccoli flowers, cabbage, parsley, peas. Grate broccoli stem, squash, cucumber, carrot, turnip. Slice kumquats.

In exact center of large plate, place large cheese ball rolled in chopped nuts. Arrange 4 prepared grapefruit sections to radiate from nut-cheese ball, giving the appearance of a star.

Around edge of plate arrange 4 lettuce cups at equal distances. Between each 2 cups place a tangerine section.

Fill lettuce cups lightly as follows:

1. grated turnip, chopped peas, with garnish of 2 slices black grape.
2. small amount grated carrot, chopped cabbage mixed with chopped parsley. Bury a small herbal cream cheese ball in this mixture.
3. grated cucumber and sliced kumquats.
4. grated squash, chopped and grated broccoli. Bury a small herbal cream cheese ball in this mixture.

SUN STAR

THE SAME RECIPE SIMPLIFIED FOR YOUR HOME

INGREDIENTS

 2 *grapefruits*
 1 *persimmon*
 1 *green pepper*
 1 *cup herbal cream cheese mixture*
 ¼ *cup pistachio nuts*
 3 *acorn squash*
 2 *large white turnips*
16 *small lettuce cups*

METHOD

Peel grapefruit and remove 8 perfect sections. Cut free from white membrane. Slice thin sections from persimmon. Cut thin strips of green pepper. Cut gash into fat edge of each grapefruit section and insert persimmon section. On each side of persimmon section, place strips of green pepper.

Make 4 large herbal cheese balls and roll in chopped pistachio nuts.

Grate acorn squash. Peel turnip and grate.

In center of the plate, place large herbal cheese ball which has been rolled in nuts. Arrange 4 prepared grapefruit sections to radiate from cheese ball giving the appearance of a star.

Around edge of plate place 4 lettuce cups at equal distances.

Fill cups lightly as follows:

1. grated acorn squash, garnished with very little white turnip.
2. squash and turnip well mixed together.
3. turnip garnished with a little squash.
4. squash and turnip well mixed together.

IMPERIAL GARDEN

(4 INDIVIDUAL MATIÈRE VIVANTE PLATES)

AS PREPARED IN THE ZURICH ROOM

INGREDIENTS

  2 *medium size cantaloupes*
  2 *large grapefruits*
  1 *cup blueberries*
  4 *pieces chicory*
 12 *fresh dates*
 ½ *orange, juice and rind*
  4 *walnuts*
 ½ *pound peas*
 ¼ *pound lima beans*
  1 *crooked neck squash*
  1 *beet*
  1 *zucchini*
  1 *carrot*
 ½ *summer squash*
 ½ *turnip*
 ¼ *tomato*
  8 *black grapes*
 16 *small lettuce cups*
  4 *herbal cream cheese balls*

METHOD

Cut cantaloupes in half and peel. Peel grapefruit and separate into perfect pieces, free of all membrane. Wash blueberries. Cut chicory into pieces. Grind dates and mix with juice and rind of ½ orange. Form into 4 balls. Chop walnuts, peas, lima beans. Grate crooked neck squash, beets, zucchini, carrot, summer squash, turnip. Make 4 small slices of the tomato.

In center of large plate, place half cantaloupe. Fill center lightly with cut chicory and sections of grapefruit. Arrange grapefruit sections to turn outward like flower petals. Scatter blueberries over top.

Place 4 lettuce cups around edge of plate at equal distances. Fill lettuce cups lightly as follows:

1. grated crooked neck squash, chopped peas, topped with three slices of black grapes.
2. herbal cream cheese ball, grated broccoli, grated beets.
3. grated summer squash, chopped lima beans, garnished with tomato slice.
4. grated turnip, date ball, grated carrot, chopped walnuts.

IMPERIAL GARDEN

(4 SERVINGS)

THE SAME RECIPE SIMPLIFIED FOR YOUR HOME

INGREDIENTS

2 *medium size cantaloupes*

2 *large grapefruits*

1 *cup blueberries*

2 *leaves of lettuce*

1 *large zucchini*

2 *large carrots*

16 *small lettuce cups*

8 *small herbal cream cheese balls*

2 *tablespoons chopped nuts*

METHOD

Cut cantaloupes in half, peel. Peel grapefruit, separate into perfect sections, be sure all membrane is removed. Wash blueberries. Cut 2 leaves of lettuce fine. Wash zucchini and grate. Wash carrots and grate.

In center of a large plate, put the cantaloupe half. Fill center lightly with shredded lettuce. Then fill with grapefruit sections arranged so they turn outward like flower petals. Scatter blueberries over top.

Place 4 lettuce cups around edge of plate at equal distances.

Fill cups lightly as follows:

1. herbal cream cheese ball covered with zucchini.
2. carrot garnished with walnuts.
3. herbal cream cheese ball, covered with zucchini and carrot which has been well mixed.
4. zucchini with a topping of carrot.

PEACH SOLSTICE

(4 INDIVIDUAL MATIÈRE VIVANTE PLATES)

AS PREPARED IN THE ZURICH ROOM

INGREDIENTS

4 *large peaches*
12 *cherries with stems*
¼ *cup herbal cream cheese mixture*
½ *young cabbage*
1 *small pineapple*
4 *radishes*
1 *green pepper*
1 *small grapefruit*
1 *small piece chicory*
1 *zucchini*
1 *yellow squash*
1 *small white squash*
¼ *pound green peas*
¼ *pound lima beans*
4 *strawberries*
4 *green grapes*
4 *large lettuce cups*
4 *herbal cream cheese balls*
12 *small romaine leaves*

METHOD

Peel peaches. Cut in half. Cover with fruit juice. Chill until ready to use. Pit cherries, leaving on stems. Stuff with herbal cream cheese mixture. Chop cabbage. Cut pineapple into fine cubes. Slice radishes, unpeeled, into fine discs. Chop green pepper fine. Remove sections from grapefruit. Using scissors, cut chicory into fine pieces and shape romaine leaves to point at both ends. Grate unpeeled zucchini, yellow squash, white squash. Chop green peas and lima beans. Hull strawberries and slice crosswise. Slice unpeeled green grapes.

Using 2 perfect firm lettuce leaves, form a cup and place it in center of large plate. Place a layer of chopped cabbage in the cup and on this arrange diced pineapple and 2 sections of grapefruit. Over this lay the 2 peach halves, one with concave side turned down, the other with concave side turned up, and filled lightly with one herbal cream cheese ball. Garnish this central lettuce cup with chopped green pepper and radish discs and a small piece of cut chicory.

Arrange 3 romaine cups about the outer part of the plate at equal distances from each other. Between each 2 romaine cups, place a stuffed cherry with its stem.

Fill the romaine cups lightly as follows:

1. arrange grated zucchini, and on top place 3 slices of strawberry.
2. fill with grated yellow squash, a few chopped green peas, and 4 slices of green grapes.
3. fill with grated white squash and chopped lima beans.

183

PEACH SOLSTICE

(4 SERVINGS)

THE SAME RECIPE SIMPLIFIED FOR YOUR HOME

INGREDIENTS

 4 *large peaches*
12 *cherries with stems*
 1 *cup herbal cream cheese mixture*
½ *young cabbage*
 1 *small pineapple*
 2 *radishes*
 3 *large carrots*
 1 *large white squash*
 4 *large lettuce cups*
12 *whole pistachio nuts*
12 *small lettuce cups*

METHOD

Peel peaches, cut in half, cover with fruit juice. Chill until ready to use. Pit cherries, leaving stems on. Stuff with herbal cream cheese mixture. Make four balls out of remainder of cheese. Chop cabbage. Cut pineapple into fine cubes. Slice radishes very thin. Scrub carrots and grate. Scrub white squash and grate.

In center of a large plate place the large lettuce cups. Fill with chopped cabbage and diced pineapple. On top lay the two peach halves, one concave side up and the other with concave side down. Place a cheese ball in the peach which is concave side up and stick whole pistachios that have been blanched into it. Garnish with sliced radishes.

Place the 3 lettuce cups at equal distances on the plate. Between each 2 cups place a cherry.

Fill the cups lightly as follows:

1. grated carrot.
2. grated squash.
3. combination of squash and carrot.

STRAWBERRY GARDEN

(4 INDIVIDUAL MATIÈRE VIVANTE PLATES)

AS PREPARED IN THE ZURICH ROOM

INGREDIENTS

1 *small pineapple*
¼ *cup blanched almonds*
1 *pint large strawberries*
1 *grapefruit*
1 *small piece of prickly pear*
12 *dates*
¼ *cup herbal cream cheese mixture*
¼ *pound lima beans*
½ *head of cabbage*
¼ *pound peas*
1 *cucumber*
8 *radishes*
½ *yellow turnip*
1 *acorn squash*
1 *summer squash*
4 *large lettuce cups*
12 *small lettuce cups*

METHOD

Peel and dice pineapple. Slice almonds into slender strips. Wash and hull strawberries. Peel grapefruit and separate into perfect sections. Cut prickly pear into 4 small pieces. Into each strawberry stick 4 or 5 almond strips. Stuff dates with herbal cream cheese mixture.

Chop lima beans, cabbage, peas. Grate cucumber, radishes, turnip, acorn squash, summer squash.

In center of large plate, place large lettuce cup. Cover bottom with chopped cabbage, then fill with diced pineapple. Across top lay 2 grapefruit sections. Arrange 4 prepared strawberries on top of all.

Place 3 lettuce cups around edge of plate at equal distances. Between each 2 lettuce cups place a stuffed date.

Fill lettuce cups lightly as follows:

1. grated cucumber and grated radish.
2. grated turnip, grated acorn squash, chopped peas.
3. grated crooked neck squash, chopped lima beans, garnished with small piece of prickly pear.

STRAWBERRY GARDEN

(4 SERVINGS)

THE SAME RECIPE SIMPLIFIED FOR YOUR HOME

INGREDIENTS

1 *small pineapple*
¼ *cup blanched almonds*
1 *pint large strawberries*
½ *cup herbal cream cheese mixture*
½ *head of cabbage*
2 *cucumbers*
1 *beet*
1 *large white turnip*
4 *large lettuce cups*
12 *small lettuce cups*
12 *dates*

METHOD

Peel and dice pineapple. Slice almonds into slender strips. Wash and hull strawberries. Into each strawberry stick 4 or 5 almond strips. Stuff dates with herbal cream cheese mixture. Chop cabbage.

Grate cucumbers, beet, and white turnip. (Peel beet and turnip first.)

In center of large plate place a large lettuce cup. Cover bottom with chopped cabbage, then fill with diced pineapple. Arrange 4 prepared strawberries on top of mound.

Place 3 lettuce cups around edge of plate at equal distances. Between each 2 cups place a stuffed date.

Fill cups lightly as follows:

1. cucumber.
2. beet with a garnish of white turnip.
3. turnip with a garnish of beet.

SUN SHAFT

AS PREPARED IN THE ZURICH ROOM

INGREDIENTS

1 *large pineapple*
1 *large grapefruit*
1 *large orange*
½ *prickly pear*
4 *large strawberries*
½ *cup herbal cream cheese mixture*
4 *fresh dates*
½ *pound peas*
½ *cup raw spinach*
1 *small cauliflower*
¼ *pound lima beans*
1 *cucumber*
1 *acorn squash*
1 *yellow squash*
4 *pieces chicory*
8 *lettuce cups*

METHOD

Peel pineapple and remove eyes. Slice lengthwise into quarters, leaving a few spines intact on end of each quarter. Peel grapefruit and separate into perfect sections; free of white membrane. Peel orange. Cut crosswise into slices 2 inches thick. Then cut each slice in half along the diameter. Cut gash in each slice and insert chopped peas into the gash.

Cut prickly pear into very small pieces. Wash strawberries, leaving hull intact. Split and insert herbal cream cheese mixture. Pit date and stuff with herbal cheese.

Chop peas, spinach, cauliflower, lima beans. Grate cucumber, acorn squash, yellow squash.

Along upper edge of pineapple quarter lay 2 sections grapefruit, alternating with 2 prepared sections orange. Place prepared pineapple across large plate. At one end, a little aside, place a stuffed strawberry on a bed of cut chicory, at the other end a stuffed date. Place a lettuce cup on each side of the pineapple.

Fill lettuce cups lightly as follows:

1. grated cucumber, grated acorn squash, chopped spinach.
2. grated yellow squash, chopped cauliflower, chopped lima beans, and garnish of small piece prickly pear.

SUN SHAFT

(4 SERVINGS)

THE SAME RECIPE SIMPLIFIED FOR YOUR HOME

INGREDIENTS

- 1 *large pineapple*
- 1 *large grapefruit*
- 1 *large orange*
- 4 *large strawberries*
- ½ *cup herbal cream cheese mixture*
- 2 *acorn squash*
- 2 *white turnips*
- 4 *baby lettuce cups*
- 8 *medium size lettuce cups*
- 1 *tablespoon chopped walnuts*

METHOD

Peel pineapple and remove eyes. Slice lengthwise into quarters, leaving a few spines intact on end of each quarter. Peel grapefruit and separate into perfect sections; free of all white membrane. Peel orange and separate into perfect sections. Leave hulls on strawberries, wash, partially cut through middle lengthwise and stuff with herbal cream cheese mixture. Make 4 balls of remaining cheese mixture. Grate acorn squash. Peel turnip and grate.

In center of a plate lay one of the quarters of pineapple. Along upper edge lay 2 grapefruit sections alternating with 2 orange sections. At the base of pineapple on the baby lettuce cup, place the stuffed strawberry. At spine end on one side place a cheese ball. Place 1 lettuce cup on either side of pineapple.

Fill lightly as follows:

1. turnip garnished with a little squash.
2. squash garnished with walnuts.

GAUGUIN SUNBURST

(4 INDIVIDUAL MATIÈRE VIVANTE PLATES)

AS PREPARED IN THE ZURICH ROOM

INGREDIENTS

24 *fresh dates*
3 *almonds*
rind and juice of ½ *orange*
2 *pieces of chicory*
4 *fresh apricots*
12 *medium size prunes*
12 *walnuts*
½ *small head cabbage*
½ *bunch watercress*
¼ *small head cauliflower*
¼ *small white squash*
1 *small crooked neck squash*
1 *carrot*
1 *small zucchini*
2 *small beets*
12 *small lettuce cups*

METHOD

Pit dates, blanch almonds. Put dates and almonds through grinder. Grate orange and squeeze. Combine ground dates, almonds, orange rind, and juice. Mix well. Divide into 4 equal parts. Cut chicory. Cut apricots into quarters. Stuff prunes with walnuts. Chop cabbage, watercress. Grate cauliflower, white squash, crooked neck squash, carrot, zucchini, beets.

Mold a ring of the date mixture in center of large plate. In center, place cut chicory and 4 apricot sections. Around edge of plate, place 3 lettuce cups at equal distances. Between each 2 cups, place stuffed prunes.

Fill lettuce cups lightly as follows:

1. grated cauliflower, grated white squash mixed, and grated beets.
2. grated zucchini, grated carrot and chopped cabbage.
3. grated crooked neck squash and chopped watercress.

GAUGUIN SUNBURST

(4 SERVINGS)

THE SAME RECIPE SIMPLIFIED FOR YOUR HOME

INGREDIENTS

36 *fresh dates*
 3 *almonds*
   juice and rind of ½ orange
   leaves of lettuce
 1 *whole orange*
12 *walnuts*
 2 *small white squash*
 3 *large beets*
12 *small lettuce cups*

METHOD

Pit dates, blanch almonds. Put 24 dates and almonds through a meat grinder. Mix with juice and grated orange rind. Mix well. Divide into 4 equal parts. Cut lettuce leaves very fine. Peel and section whole orange. Stuff 12 remaining dates with walnuts. Grate squash. Peel beets and grate.

Mold a ring of the date mixture in center of a large plate. In center place the shredded lettuce. Fill with orange sections. Around edge of plate put the 3 lettuce cups; between each 2 cups place a stuffed date.

Fill cups lightly as follows:

1. grated squash garnished with beets.
2. beets garnished with white squash.
3. mixture of beets and squash, well blended.

SWIRLING SUNLIGHT

(4 INDIVIDUAL MATIÈRE VIVANTE PLATES)

AS PREPARED IN THE ZURICH ROOM

INGREDIENTS

16 *cherry tomatoes*

½ *honeydew melon*

1 *grapefruit*

16 *lettuce cups*

4 *pieces chicory*

1 *cup herbal cream cheese mixture*

1 *small zucchini*

¼ *pomegranate*

¼ *cup pistachio nuts*

1 *beet*

½ *turnip*

1 *small crooked neck squash*

¼ *cabbage*

¼ *bunch parsley*

1 *carrot*

1 *cucumber*

METHOD

Peel honeydew. Cut 16 crescent-shaped sections. Grind pistachio nuts. Peel grapefruit and separate into perfect sections, free of all white membrane. Remove seeds from pomegranate; cut chicory. Clean cherry tomatoes. Chop cabbage and parsley. Grate zucchini, turnip, beet, crooked neck squash, carrot, cucumber.

In center of large plate, make ring of 4 cherry tomatoes held in place by herbal cream cheese mixture border. In center of cherry tomato ring, place chicory and grapefruit sections. Sprinkle pistachio nuts over grapefruit.

From each cherry tomato, place a honeydew melon crescent to extend toward edge of plate, having the 4 crescents lie parallel.

Between each 2 melon crescents, place a lettuce cup.

Fill lettuce cups lightly as follows:

1. grated zucchini, garnished with pomegranate seeds.
2. grated turnip, garnished with grated beets.
3. grated crooked neck squash, grated cucumber.
4. grated carrot, mixed chopped cabbage and chopped parsley.

SWIRLING SUNLIGHT

(4 SERVINGS)

THE SAME RECIPE SIMPLIFIED FOR YOUR HOME

INGREDIENTS

1 *honeydew melon*
¼ *cup pistachio nuts*
4 *lettuce leaves*
1 *bunch broccoli*
3 *large carrots*
16 *cherry tomatoes*
1 *cup herbal cream cheese mixture*
16 *small lettuce cups*

METHOD

Peel honeydew. From one half cut 16 crescent shaped sections. Grind pistachio nuts. The remaining half of the honeydew, peel and dice. Cut 4 lettuce leaves very fine. Grate stems of broccoli, chop flowers and mix them together. Scrape carrots and grate.

In center of a large plate make a ring of 4 cherry tomatoes, held in place by herbal cream cheese mixture border. In center of ring place the shredded lettuce. Fill center with diced honeydew. Sprinkle pistachio nuts over top.

From each cherry tomato lay a honeydew melon crescent to extend towards edge of plate having 4 crescents lying parallel. Between each 2 crescents place a lettuce cup.

Fill lettuce cups lightly as follows:

1. broccoli garnished with carrot.
2. mixture of broccoli and carrot.
3. carrot garnished with broccoli.
4. mixture of broccoli and carrot.

GLITTERING PEAR

(4 INDIVIDUAL MATIÈRE VIVANTE PLATES)

AS PREPARED IN THE ZURICH ROOM

INGREDIENTS

 4 *large bartlett pears*
 1 *cup herbal cream cheese mixture*
   a few spears chicory
 8 *cherry tomatoes*
 4 *large strawberries*
 8 *black grapes*
   a few peas
   a few lima beans
 2 *pieces parsley*
 1 *zucchini*
 1 *yellow squash*
 1 *white squash*
 ½ *turnip*
 2 *tablespoons ground pistachio nuts*
16 *small lettuce cups*

METHOD

Peel pears, then cut each in quarters lengthwise. Sprinkle pears with citrus fruit juice. Make 4 large balls of herbal cream cheese mixture. Cut chicory fine. Cut cherry tomatoes in half. Slice strawberries and slice black grapes. Shell peas and limas and chop fine. Chop parsley.

Grate zucchini, yellow squash, white squash, and turnips.

In center of large plate, place a little cut chicory, using this as a bed. On it place a cheese ball. Around this ball group 4 cherry tomato halves. From this center radiate 4 quarter pieces of pear and on one edge of each piece put a little chopped pistachio. Group 4 lettuce cups around edge of plate.

Fill lightly as follows:

1. zucchini, 2 slices of strawberries.
2. turnip, walnut, 2 slices of black grapes.
3. yellow squash and peas.
4. white squash, limas, parsley.

GLITTERING PEAR

THE SAME RECIPE SIMPLIFIED FOR YOUR HOME

(4 SERVINGS)

INGREDIENTS

4 *large barlett pears*
1 *cup herbal cream cheese mixture*
2 *tablespoons ground pistachio nuts*
2 *leaves lettuce*
1 *large yellow squash*
1 *large zucchini*
2 *sprigs parsley*
16 *small lettuce cups*

METHOD

Peel pears, cut in fourths lengthwise, soak in fruit juice. Make 4 large balls of herbal cream cheese mixture, roll in pistachio nuts. Cut the 2 leaves of lettuce into fine shreds. Grate squash and zucchini. Chop parsley.

In center of a large plate, make a small bed of lettuce shreds. On it place the cheese ball. Group the 4 pieces of pear so they look like a flower.

Place 4 lettuce cups around and fill as follows:

1. zucchini garnished with squash.
2. squash garnished with parsley.
3. squash and zucchini mixed.
4. squash and zucchini mixed.

GRAPES IN SUNLIGHT

(4 INDIVIDUAL MATIÈRE VIVANTE PLATES)

AS PREPARED IN THE ZURICH ROOM

INGREDIENTS

1 *pound large black grapes*
1 *cup herbal cream cheese mixture*
8 *very small spears of endive*
2 *tablespoons ground pistachio nuts*
½ *persimmon*
6 *cherry tomatoes*
1 *head romaine*
1 *small pineapple*
1 *zucchini*
1 *small yellow squash*
1 *small carrot*
½ *white squash*
 a few lima beans
2 *pieces parsley*
¼ *head cabbage*
4 *large lettuce cups*

METHOD

Divide the grapes into 4 small clusters. With a sharp knife remove seeds and stuff with herbal cream cheese mixture. The grapes remain intact on the stems. Stuff endive spears with chopped pistachio nuts. Make 4 slices of the persimmon. Slice cherry tomatoes. With scissors trim romaine, making cups. Peel and dice pineapple.

Grate zucchini, yellow squash, carrot, and white squash. Chop lima beans, parsley, and cabbage very fine.

In center of a large plate place a large lettuce cup. Fill lightly with chopped cabbage and then with diced pineapple. Over the top sprinkle grated carrot. On top of mound lay the grape cluster. Group 3 romaine cups around plate and between 2 place the endive spears.

Fill the cups lightly as follows:

1. yellow squash, chopped lima beans, a very little parsley.
2. zucchini and 2 slices of cherry tomato.
3. white squash and a slice of persimmon.

GRAPES IN SUNLIGHT

(4 SERVINGS)

THE SAME RECIPE SIMPLIFIED FOR YOUR HOME

INGREDIENTS

½ head cabbage
1 small pineapple
1 pound grapes
1 cup herbal cream cheese mixture
1 carrot
1 zucchini
1 yellow squash
4 large lettuce cups
12 small lettuce cups
2 tablespoons ground pistachio nuts

METHOD

Chop cabbage very fine. Peel and dice pineapple. Divide grapes into 4 bunches and stuff with herbal cream cheese mixture.

Grate carrot, zucchini, and squash.

In center of a large plate place a large lettuce cup. Fill lightly with cabbage, then pineapple and sprinkle a few grated carrots over the top. On top of this place a stuffed-grape cluster.

Around the outside of plate place 3 lettuce cups.

Fill lightly as follows:

1. zucchini garnished with a little carrot.
2. yellow squash garnished with pistachio nuts.
3. zucchini and squash well blended.

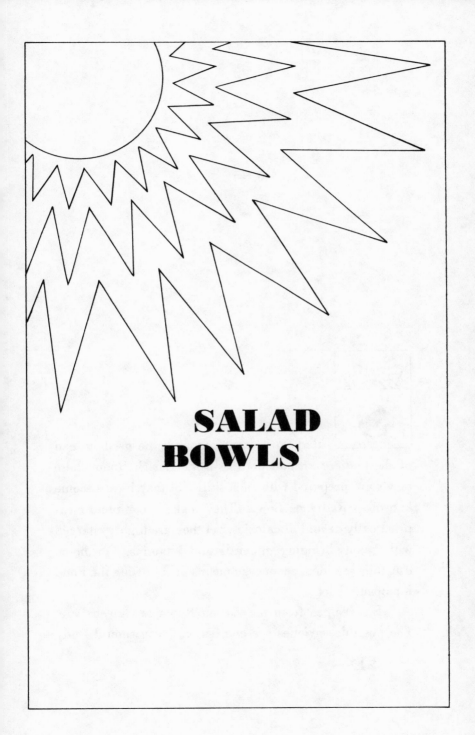

SALAD
BOWLS

Salad bowls can frequently be used instead of the *matière vivante* plates. In the Zurich Room these bowls are prepared with such skill that they have become known as Radiance Bowls. They make a complete meal practically devoid of calories, yet they are highly charged with beauty-bringing minerals and vitamins. For home use, they are ideal as an easy means of following the Food for Beauty Diet.

Six recipes from the Zurich Room are given here. The possible varieties are endless, and you should study your markets and then invent your own health- and vitality-bringing bowls. They are perfect food—in looks, in taste, and in essential elements.

The bowls can be purchased at low cost at any hardware store. Serve with one of the dressings given in an earlier chapter.

FRUIT RADIANCE SALAD BOWL I

(INDIVIDUAL)

AS PREPARED IN THE ZURICH ROOM

INGREDIENTS

¼ *head lettuce*
½ *head endive*
½ *orange*
½ *grapefruit*
½ *cup cantaloupe*
½ *cup diced pineapple*
1 *sprig watercress*
4 *Belgian or large black grapes*

METHOD

Line bowl with lettuce, then endive. Peel orange and grapefruit and cut in very careful sections so that membrane is all removed. Fill bowl with fruit so orange sections and cantaloupe are opposite each other; in center, put a sprig of watercress. Decorate with 4 Belgian or large black grapes.

FRUIT RADIANCE
SALAD BOWL I

(INDIVIDUAL)

THE SAME RECIPE SIMPLIFIED FOR YOUR HOME

INGREDIENTS

¼ *head lettuce*

4 *leaves of romaine*

4 *pieces of chicory*

⅓ *cup diced cantaloupe*

⅓ *cup diced honeydew*

⅓ *cup diced pineapple*

1 *fresh fig*

4 *large cherries with stems on*

   sprig of watercress

4 *filberts*

⅓ *grapefruit*

METHOD

Line bowl with lettuce, then romaine and chicory. Fill bowl with fruit so that cantaloupe and honeydew are opposite. On top put slices of fresh fig. In center put a sprig of watercress and at the 4 corners of bowl the cherries, which have been stuffed with nuts.

FRUIT RADIANCE SALAD BOWL II

(INDIVIDUAL)

INGREDIENTS

¼ *head lettuce*
4 *leaves romaine*
4 *pieces chicory*
⅓ *cup diced pears*
½ *cup diced pineapple*
⅓ *cup diced watermelon*
½ *diced honeydew*
1 *sprig watercress*
   a few blueberries or raspberries

METHOD

Line bowl with lettuce. Put in 4 romaine leaves and 4 pieces of chicory so they protrude over side of bowl. On 2 opposite sides fill bowl with pear and pineapple. On 2 other sides put watermelon and honeydew. In center put a sprig of watercress. Over top sprinkle a few blueberries or raspberries.

VEGETABLE RADIANCE
SALAD BOWL

(INDIVIDUAL)

INGREDIENTS

2 *pieces celery*
1 *carrot*
¼ *cucumber*
½ *tomato*
¼ *head lettuce*
4 *leaves romaine*
4 *pieces chicory*
1 *radish*
1 *sprig watercress*

METHOD

Cut celery and carrot in very thin julienne strips, put in ice water so they become crisp. Take a fork and run it down side of cucumber and then cut in very thin slices. Do not peel cucumber. Put cucumber in salted ice water. Peel tomato and cut in eighths.

Line bowl with lettuce, then romaine, then chicory. Put carrot on one side, celery on the other; between put slices of cucumber. On top put 4 sections of tomato and a sprig of watercress in center. Over all scatter a few thin slices of radish.

Individual raw fruit and vegetable salads can be used at times in place of the salad bowl. But the same delicacy and freshness must be sought. Furthermore there must be the welcome absence of fussiness and overdecoration. The following directions are very simple, being meant more as guides than as specific recipes. Often you will have fresh raw fruits and vegetables in your refrigerator; they can be used in place of the ingredients suggested here.

STRAWBERRIES IN CLOVER

Arrange a bed of crisp watercress in center of plate. Sprinkle with finely sliced celery and thinly cut almonds. Arrange hulled strawberries on top. Sprinkle with French dressing and serve with fresh cottage cheese mixed with chopped parsley and chives.

PINEAPPLE WITH BEAN SPROUTS

Make a French dressing of lime juice, pineapple juice, and selected vegetable oil.

Peel pineapple, core, and cut lengthwise into thin slices. Arrange lettuce leaf on plate, place a shallow layer of bean sprouts in bottom and lay a few pineapple slices on top. Garnish with herbal cream cheese ball and finely chopped mint. Serve with special French dressing.

PERSIMMON CHALICE

In center of plate make a bed of lettuce. On it place a persimmon which has been cut down in quarters so that it looks like a flower. Fill the center with a small herbal cream cheese ball which has been rolled in chopped peas.

Serve with lime French dressing.

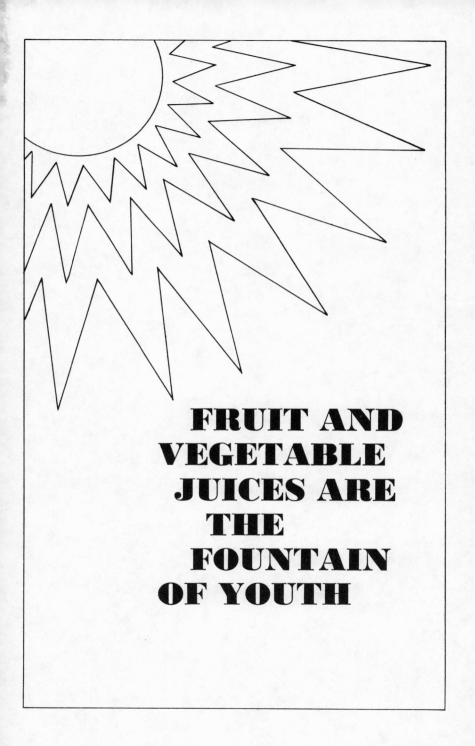

FRUIT AND VEGETABLE JUICES ARE THE FOUNTAIN OF YOUTH

The modern fruit and vegetable juice extractor is as necessary to any household as the kitchen stove. Wherever you find a lovely and vital woman, you will find a fresh fruit or vegetable juice enthusiast.

Any woman who is determined to profit by the sunlight-nutrition theory of modern diet should go to the nearest good store and study the various types of fruit and vegetable juice extractors on the market. Her choice will depend somewhat on the amount of money she cares to spend. Some juice extractors are operated electrically, others by hand. She alone can decide how large a machine she needs for herself and her family and how much she can afford to pay. It is important to study the mechanism of these various pressers and to decide in advance whether or not they can be kept clean easily. Remember, they will be in daily use in all diets.

This is as good a time as any to suggest at least one day of liquid dieting in the month. Not only will a liquid day materially aid in reducing your weight without injury, but it will also do much to remove any toxins from your body. It will be a day of very few calories, but the important thing to remember is that by using a variety of fruit and vegetable juices on this liquid day, you will in no way lessen your regular intake of essential minerals and vitamins.

Combined with a reasonable amount of exercise, the following liquid day may cause you to lose as many as 3 pounds in 24 hours. Unless your own physician has advised you against it, there is no danger to the normally healthy and somewhat overweight woman in this one day of liquids only, plus some degree of physical exercise.

The following liquid day schedule contains only 428 calories.

    8 A.M.—8 oz. orange and lemon juice mixed with
              herbal or China tea
11 A.M.—8 oz. vegetable juice
    2 P.M.—8 oz. mixed fruit juice,
              small helping of garden hors d'oeuvres

228

5 P.M.—8 oz. of fresh tomato juice

8 P.M.—8 oz. of grapefruit juice

11 P.M., or at retiring—one 5 oz. glass of butter-milk

Recipes for fruit and vegetable combinations used here are given later in this chapter.

If coffee is so important to you that its sudden elimination from the diet will upset you, include a cup of black coffee with the 8 A.M. juice and also a demitasse with the 8 P.M. juice. If possible, however, avoid coffee while on this diet.

The liquid day of mixed fruit and vegetable juices was worked out for the patrons of the Zurich Room, who combined it with their regular diet of raw fruits and vegetables. It is not only detoxicating, but it also rests the digestive tract and produces a feeling of freshness and physical cleanliness. One day in a month is such a little time to give to the rebuilding of youthfulness. You must set aside a definite day on your beauty calendar and not let it go by without this internal bath in the modern fountain of youth.

Perhaps your diet has for a long time been so wrong that your system needs a sterner treatment. You may need a special 2 to 8 day liquid diet worked out by a noted physician to eliminate poisons from the system. Whether you need follow it the full 8 days or less, will depend on how poisoned your system has become through bad eating or other forms of overindulgence. You, yourself, will have to determine its length according to the severity of your case.

Two schedules are given. One is for the first half of this liquid diet. The second schedule is for the second half of the diet. For example, if you go on the diet for 4 days, follow the first schedule for the first 2 days and then continue with the second schedule the last 2 days.

In the first column is the schedule for the first half of the diet, whether you continue it for 2 or 8 days.

7 A.M. —2 glasses lemon water (juice ½ lemon to 1 glass water) drink without stopping
8 A.M. —juice 1 grapefruit
10 A.M. —2 glasses lemon water
12 NOON—juice 1 grapefruit
2 P.M. —2 glasses lemon water
4 P.M. —juice 1 grapefruit
6 P.M. —2 glasses lemon water
8 P.M. —juice 1 grapefruit

In the second column in the schedule for the second half of the diet, whether you continue it for 2 or 8 days.

7 A.M. —2 glasses lemon water
8 A.M. —1 glass milk
10 A.M. —2 glasses lemon water
12 NOON—1 glass milk
2 P.M. —1 glass milk

230

4 P.M. —2 glasses lemon water
6 P.M. —1 glass milk
8 P.M. —1 glass milk

The use of fresh juices in American homes increases steadily as it becomes understood that they are delicious sources of vitamins. When various juices are combined, the result is not only novelty but also a vitamin balance. In the Zurich Room, many unusual combinations were developed and the cherished recipes are here given for the first time.

The following recipes are for fruit and vegetable juice combinations made famous in the Zurich Room. They were used in the liquid day described earlier in this paragraph. They are to be sipped slowly, always.

VEGETABLE CASCADE

2 *cups spinach juice*
3 *cups tomato juice*
3 *tablespoons carrot juice*
3 *tablespoons celery juice*
¼ *teaspoon salt*

TOMATO CELERY GOBLET

4 *cups tomato juice*
½ *cup celery juice*
1 *teaspoon salt*

JADE COCKTAIL

4 *cups grapefruit juice*
1 *cup spinach juice*
¼ *cup watercress juice*
pinch salt

SPRING GOBLET

2 *cups spinach juice*
2½ *cups grapefruit juice*
¾ *cup orange or lime juice*
a little pineapple honey
pinch salt

232

BLUEBERRY GOBLET

1 *box blueberries*
1 *cup orange juice*
1 *cup pineapple juice*
⅓ *cup lime juice*
  pinch salt

LIQUID JADE

2 *cups honeydew melon juice*
1 *cup pineapple juice*
⅓ *cup lime juice*
½ *teaspoon salt*

WATERMELON GOBLET

3 *cups watermelon juice (about ⅛ melon)*
1½ *cups grapefruit juice*
1 *tablespoon lime juice*
1 *teaspoon lemon juice*

CORAL GOBLET

4 *cups grapefruit juice*
8 *teaspoons radish juice*
½ *teaspoon salt*

APRICOT COCONUT GOBLET

½ *cup fresh coconut milk*
2½ *cups orange juice*
1¾ *cups apricot juice*
2 *tablespoons lime juice*
pinch salt

CORONATION GOBLET

2 *cups grapefruit juice*
1 *cup raspberry juice*
1 *cup green grape juice*
pinch salt

YOUNGBERRY GOBLET

1 *cup youngberry juice*
4 *cups grapefruit juice*
2 *cups pineapple juice*

234

TROPICAL GOBLET

4 *cups pineapple juice*
1 *cup orange juice*
2 *teaspoons lime juice*
1 *teaspoon honey*
   pinch salt

TAHITIAN COCKTAIL

2 *cups rhubarb juice*
2 *cups pineapple juice*
1 *tablespoon lime juice*
1 *tablespoon honey*
½ *cup fresh strawberry juice*

PINEAPPLE-MINT CASCADE

1 *cup pineapple juice*
2 *cups rhubarb juice*
½ *ounce mint juice*
   a little pineapple honey
   pinch salt

APPLE-LIME CASCADE

(1 quart)

3½   *cups fresh apple juice*
½   *cup fresh pineapple juice*
   juice 4 limes
1   *tablespoon honey*

CRANBERRY-PINEAPPLE CASCADE

(1 quart)

3   *cups fresh cranberry juice*
1   *cup fresh pineapple juice*
   juice 2 limes
1   *tablespoon honey*

Dessert is a dreaded and fascinating word to women who long to lose their "too, too solid flesh." But I think that is because so many Americans have not learned to appreciate the continental habit of serving fresh fruit for dessert. In this country, rich puddings, pastries, and sweet, creamy mixtures are the more usual desserts and of course they carry hundreds of unneeded calories which will turn into excess weight.

In all the Food for Beauty Diets, raw fruit is served for dessert. Apples, pears, grapes, melon, peaches, berries in season, on down through the orchard and garden

236

treasury, appear at the end of the meal to add a final gift of minerals and vitamins to the beauty-hungry woman.

But those fruits can be served in attractive arrangements as well as whole. The Fruit Glacier, an innovation which delighted visitors to the Zurich Room, can be used in your own home to give fruit desserts not only pleasant variations but also unusual beauty.

This Fruit Glacier dessert consists of an assortment of fresh fruits arranged on a tray of ice; this tray is called a Fruit Glacier. It is a very simple matter to arrange requiring no more than any ordinary waterproof tray with slightly raised edges.

On the bottom, place two folded napkins to absorb water from melting ice. Then spread a layer of cracked ice or ice cubes over the napkins. Decorate the ice with large green leaves around the edges. Use two or more combinations of fruit for each tray. The following sample combinations have proved most popular and will suggest many others for you to try.

1. Crescents of ripe honeydew melon dipped in ground pistachio nuts. Arranged on ice bed with large unhulled strawberries.
2. Spears of fresh pineapple with spines left on for handle. The sharp edge is cut into a groove, that groove is filled with fresh raspberries. Blackberries can be used, also.
3. Clusters of cherries with stems (3) tied to-

237

gether. Arranged on ice bed with pineapple balls rolled in freshly grated coconut.

4. Fresh figs, sliced to open slightly, stuffed with cream cheese and preserved ginger.

5. Perfect navel orange sections rolled in freshly grated coconut. Arranged on ice bed with clusters of black grapes.

6. Alternate clusters of large green grapes and large black grapes. Arranged on ice bed with cantaloupe balls rolled in ground pistachio nuts.

7. Perfect tangerine sections. Arranged on ice bed with pineapple balls rolled in freshly grated coconut.

8. Alternated crescents of Persian melon and honeydew melon.

9. Perfect apricot halves, concave side up. Arranged on ice bed with clusters of 3 cherries, tied.

10. Perfect thin discs of bright prickly pear. Arranged on ice bed with pineapple balls.

The color and flavor contrasts and harmonies possible for the Fruit Glacier are really endless. I urge you to study your gardens and your markets and invent an endless series of beautiful desserts which will delight you and each member of your family while they overcome their cravings for pastries and puddings.

238

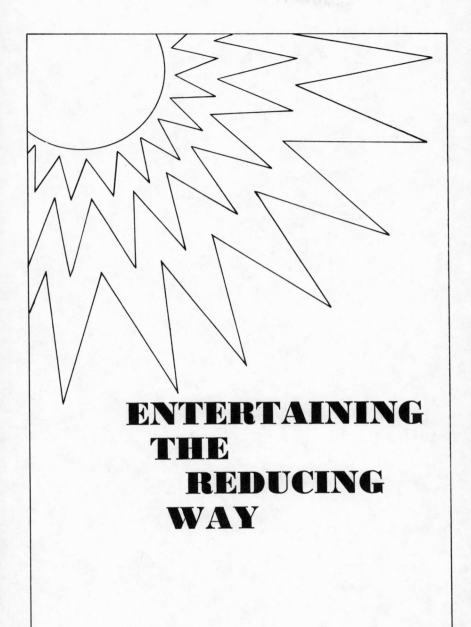

ENTERTAINING THE REDUCING WAY

Slenderness does not bar sociability. It is a simple matter to entertain your dieting friends without many calories to their day. In fact, the afternoon tea hour in the Zurich Room introduced a fashion in nonfattening sociability which you can now follow in your own home.

In the Zurich Room, a multicolored assortment of gay canapes and hors d'oeuvres appeared each afternoon to gladden the friendly hearts of dieting women who liked to meet for tea and yet not be tempted to nibble themselves back to plumpness. These deceptive mouthfuls of non-

fattening indulgences are made of raw fruits and vegetables skillfully rolled in whole wheat and other health
breads. They are usually served with fresh fruit or vegetable juices, though tea with lemon often appears. Never
does a lump of sugar or a gram of cream come to the
party.

If you are seeking ideas with which to startle and
delight your friends, I suggest that you invite them to a
Zurich Room Tea. If they, like you, are following the
Food for Beauty Diet, they will be doubly grateful for
your invitation. These canapes and hors d'oeuvres are
part of the diet and will help you increase your daily
consumption of raw fruits and vegetables.

The canapes are really rolled sandwiches cut into
slender slices. Rather than give too many specific recipes
for these rolled canapes, we will take one or two examples to show you how they are done. After that you
must continue to invent your own, using whatever vegetables or fruits appeal to you. Let us begin with a tiny
bread ring with a slice of carrot gold for its heart.

This is how it is done: Scrape a slender carrot, sizing
it down to even thickness; cut a thin slice of whole wheat
bread lengthwise of the loaf and spread it smoothly with
cream cheese, seasoning with chopped herbs. Lay the
carrot on one side of the slice and roll the bread around
it. Seal the overlapping edge with cheese, then tightly
wrap the carrot roll in wax paper and chill in the refrigerator at least three hours. Just before serving, slice
into thin rings.

Radishes, cucumbers, strips of stuffed celery can be used in the same manner.

For sweeter, nonfattening hors d'oeuvres, use fresh pineapple, pears, and other fruits. Big black meaty cherries, for example, are pitted, stuffed with cheese and rolled in cheesed bread and sliced into rings. One cherry makes four little rolled sandwiches, each of half dollar size.

Here are some more designs for your slenderizing afternoon tea. Freshly chopped fresh vegetables are laid in diagonal lines across a length of the loaf slice of bread. Spread it lightly with herb-seasoned cream cheese or nonfattening mayonnaise. Then roll the bread, chill, and slice. You get four raw vegetables in a single pinwheel: chopped green pepper, grated carrots, grated summer squash, and chopped lima beans.

To make ribbon sandwiches, use crisp garden vegetables and fresh fruit for the layer. Another idea is to take an oblong of nut bread, 5 inches long, ½ inch thick, and spread on all sides with cream cheese. Roll this in a thin slice of gluten bread. Wrap in wax paper and chill before serving.

To serve these Zurich Room delicacies, arrange them daintily on a crystal plate, together with some of the other fresh fruit and vegetable hors d'oeuvres suggested below. They are about as delicate and as charming little things to eat as any of your dieting friends ever saw at a tea party.

Serve garden hors d'oeuvres also with your Zurich

tea. They should be displayed together with the canapes on tastefully arranged dishes. Keep your variety large.

The following is a list of the hors d'oeuvres served in the Zurich Room for afternoon tea. With a little practice, you will be able to make these afternoon delicacies yourself. They combine raw fruits and vegetables in delightful tidbits for the low-caloried afternoon meal.

HORS D'OEUVRES

FRUIT

APRICOT—

Half apricot rolled in coconut
Half apricot with half walnut center

DATES—

Stuffed with cream cheese
Stuffed with green peppers
Stuffed with strawberries
Stuffed with cherries
Stuffed with watercress (chopped)
Stuffed with half walnut
Stuffed with half pecan

244

CHERRIES—

Stuffed with fresh coconut

Stuffed with herbal cheese mixture, nuts sprinkled on
top

Tied in bunches of three. Effective and unusual

FIGS—

Small sections rolled in coconut

Small sections rolled in ground pistachio nuts

Small sections rolled in ground walnuts

GRAPES—

Stuffed with herbal cream cheese mixture

Stuffed with cream cheese, nuts sprinkled on top

KUMQUATS—

Stuffed with cream cheese, ground nuts. Minced pre-
served ginger

Stuffed with date mixture

MELON—

Cantaloupe balls rolled in ground pistachio nuts

Cantaloupe balls rolled in ground walnuts

Cantaloupe balls rolled in ground almonds

Honeydew balls rolled in ground pistachio nuts

Honeydew balls rolled in ground almonds

Honeydew balls rolled in ground walnuts

245

ORANGE—

> Sections rolled in grated coconut. Simple and effective

PINEAPPLE—

> Balls rolled in grated fresh coconut
> Balls rolled in ground pistachio nuts
> Balls rolled in ground almonds
> Balls rolled in ground walnuts
> Fingers—slender spears

PRUNES—

> Stuffed with half walnut
> Stuffed with half pecan

STRAWBERRIES—

> Whole with hulls
> Split and stuffed with cream cheese. Stems intact

PLUMS—

> Half plum with half walnut for the center
> Plum sections rolled in grated coconut

AVOCADO—

> Small slice avocado, edge dipped in grated cauliflower

GARDEN VEGETABLE CUPS

LETTUCE—

Filled with grated carrot, marinated in reducing dressing

Filled with grated cucumber, marinated in reducing dressing

Filled with grated cucumber, marinated in reducing dressing and topped with grated radishes

CELERY—

Stuffed with avocado pear mixture (dusted with ground nuts)

Stuffed with grated radishes

Stuffed with chopped watercress and grated radishes

ENDIVE HEARTS—

Stuffed with avocado pear mixture and topped with grated cauliflower

Stuffed with grated radish

Stuffed with cream cheese mixture and grated zucchini

RADISHES—

Roses

SANDWICHES

NUT BREAD—

    Spread with cream cheese

    Spread with avocado pear mixture

    Topped with very thinly sliced tomato

    Spread with carrot and pineapple mixture

    Spread with parsnip and watercress mixture

    Rolled with cream cheese mixture

WHOLE WHEAT BREAD—

    Spread with cream cheese mixture with a few drops of watercress juice added

    Spread with cream cheese mixture having a celery center stuffed with chopped watercress

PEPPER SANDWICHES—

    Strips of green pepper spread with cream cheese mixture to hold

INDEX

249

250

251